WOUNDED WARRIORS

WOUNDED WARRIORS

A Soldier's Story of Healing through Birds

Robert C. Vallieres with
Jacquelyn M. Howard

Foreword by Cynthia Parsons

POTOMAC BOOKS
An imprint of the University of Nebraska Press

♾

Library of Congress
Cataloging-in-Publication Data

Vallieres, Robert C.
Wounded warriors: a soldier's story
of healing through birds / Robert C.
Vallieres with Jacquelyn M. Howard;
foreword by Cynthia Parsons.

pages   cm

ISBN 978-1-61234-582-6 (cloth : alk.
paper)—ISBN 978-1-61234-583-3 (pdf) 1.
Vallieres, Robert C.—Mental health. 2.
Post-traumatic stress disorder—Patients—
United States—Biography. 3. Brain
damage—Patients—Rehabilitation. 4. Bird
watching—Therapeutic use. 5. Veterans—
Mental health—United States—Biography.
I. Howard, Jacquelyn M. II. Title.

RC552.P67 V35 2014
616.85'2120092—dc23
[B]
2013042869

Set in Minion by Lindsey Auten.
Designed by N. Putens.

To the men and women of our United States Armed Forces—past, present, and future—and to my unit, the XVIII Airborne Corps, 175th Engineer Company, 30th Engineer Battalion, 20th Engineer Brigade.

Above all else, guard your heart, for everything you do flows from it.
~Proverbs 4:23

Contents

Foreword

*Do not fear the winds of adversity. Remember—a
kite rises against the wind rather than with it.*
~Unknown

I am Cindy Parsons and I am a Wounded Warrior mom. My son, Sergeant Shane Parsons, suffered a severe anoxic brain injury and two cardiac arrests, eventually succumbing to bilateral above-the-knee amputations. He has been my inspiration to do more with my life.

What does it mean to do "more with one's life"? How can a trauma experienced by a loved one translate into inspiration for my life, your life, or for the authors of this book—Robert, a disabled vet since 1990, and Jackie, a military contractor and biologist? What generates in us the power to rise above the injury, the insurmountable wounding; what drives the physical, biological, psychological, emotional, and life-changing reconfiguration of human pathos into a mission of witnessing to others, showing them that life does not end but changes and continues, takes us down that road less traveled, and lets us soar with instead of being grounded by severe suffering, loss, and trauma?

I, as a mom, worry about my son each and every minute of each and every day, but the worry changes into an acceptance of the way things are now and an understanding of how Shane can function moving forward, not wallowing in self-pity over why it happened to him, to me—his only parent—or to you.

Robert Vallieres, over twenty years ago, I am certain, asked these same questions, as, I am also certain, did his wife. How could this happen—one day he is alive and well and then the startling call and realization that he is not, I am not, you are not, none of us are—that life has changed in such a way that there is no circling back, ever.

My son, Shane, as a young boy always loved the outdoors. I remember vividly the time when he was five years old and ran through the kitchen excitedly repeating, "Mommy, Mommy look what I found," opening his little hands to show me a little bird he had found outside while playing. Always the typical mom, I told him to drop it outside and come back in and wash his hands. He would not but continued to unfurl his fingers and reveal to me the bird in his hand—a tiny, almost feathered baby robin. I smile knowingly to myself remembering this and am thankful he didn't do as I had hastily asked. He was always outside and always rescuing animals—turtles, more birds, small animals, anything that was in need of help and rescue. He was connected to and cared for all living things.

But most of all, he loved fishing. And, through the YMCA summer camps he attended, he became adept at identifying birds—hawks, orioles, blue jays, robins, and many others. One time when he and I were out walking, a bird came down almost in front of us and grabbed a baby rabbit. I screamed, but Shane calmly said that the bird was a hawk and just needed to eat and that is why it killed the rabbit. He stayed calm and understood the custody of creation, where some are killed so that others may eat.

I relate these memories because they give insight into Shane as a person, a soldier, and a traumatically injured and recovering veteran. During Shane's long and painful injury through stabilization and recovery, he was transferred from Walter Reed Army Medical Center (after he was infection-free and his surgeries were done) to a traumatic brain injury ward at the Veterans Administration (VA) hospital in Minneapolis for another postrecovery phase of rehabilitation.

The transfer flight was very painful and difficult for me. During the flight, Shane's pain threshold destabilized and the medics on board could not bring it back under control. The decision was made to divert the flight to the nearest airport where additional medical assistance could be provided. We touched down at an intermediary city (I cannot remember the name) and Shane was given additional medical care on board. But his pain threshold was still not stabilized. He was hurting and I hurt right alongside him. The plane took off again and we eventually landed in Minneapolis, where he was transported to the VA hospital, traumatic brain injury section.

Shane became very emotional—excessive pain brought on emotional depression and memories of what he had been through. He asked to see a priest and, because none were available, a preacher was sent in. The preacher was a godsend; he held Shane's hand, giving him physical comfort and emotional support. I left the room so that they could speak. As I remember it, this was a turning point for Shane, as he desperately needed a spiritual friend, a man of faith and of God to be with him during this crisis.

I want to emphasize that when Shane was released from Walter Reed his pain was under control, he had recovered from his surgeries and was infection-free. The unexpected turn of events on the flight to Minneapolis could not have been anticipated. As a trained emergency room nurse, I believe that the constant jarring motion and noise contributed to his pain destabilization, which in turn brought back the memory of the trauma . . . from being in Iraq and suffering the traumatic head injury through losing his legs.

But it was still hard to watch my son thrash in bed, cry for relief, tears rolling down his face—tears brought on by emotional and physical pain as well as by remembering how it all happened. Memory can be as cruel as it can be wonderful.

Shane remained under constant surveillance while at the Minneapolis facility, a total of three months.

The saving grace for Shane, and for me, was the day a Vietnam veteran with a Bronze Star and his wife came to the trauma unit for a visit. This was during the first four weeks of Shane's residence. The vet's name was Bob and he and his wife were volunteers with a raptor rehabilitation center. Once a month Bob, his wife, and a bald eagle named Harriet would drive at least an hour to visit the VA hospital. Harriet was a rehabilitated eagle who was used in therapy for wounded vets in Minneapolis.

The instant Shane was introduced to this wounded eagle he began to recover. He would smile, anticipating the next visit of Bob and Harriet, the wounded eagle that he knew understood him and what he had been through. Shane, the Vietnam vet Bob, and Harriet, the eagle who could not fly, bonded and miracles happened.

Harriet the eagle would visit only once per month, but Bob would come to see Shane more frequently. Bob would come and spend an hour with Shane behind closed doors. I never invited myself into their conversations and never asked what was said between them. The only hint of what they talked about was when Shane told me that Bob had been exposed to Agent Orange.

Why the eagle? Why Bob? I no longer ask. All I can say is this: that eagle healed Shane in ways no human possibly could, and Bob brought the eagle to Shane. One time Bob let Shane stroke the feathers on Harriet's back. Shane and the bird locked eyes and Shane said, "See, Mom, when I stare into Harriet's eyes, she understands me, understands my pain, I can see it in her eyes." Shane, Harriet, and Bob gained such trust with each other that Shane was allowed to hold and feed Harriet, which for me was both a spiritual and a real experience, life affirming life on a very profound level. Eventually, Bob and his wife invited Shane and me on a tour of the raptor center, just before Shane was released. During this tour Bob's wife told me that eagles had saved Bob's life; he has been suicidal as well.

Shane has never lost his affinity for eagles. About two years after his release from the Minneapolis hospital, while we were on a camping and rafting trip in Colorado with other wounded vets, Shane noticed an eagle following alongside the rafts. We all saw the eagle, and it followed our rafts for many miles as we drifted down the river. Shane and I are sure that the eagle knew that these rafts were full of Wounded Warriors, defenders of freedom both here and abroad, and was there as the symbol of our great country to acknowledge their sacrifice and to afford them and their families protection from above.

I see birds as a veritable moving feast of multisensory color, texture, and sound that captures our imaginations, heals our sorrows, validates our pain, and symbolizes our strength and unity as a nation and a people. Please take the time to introduce a wounded, disabled, post-traumatic vet and yourself to birds . . . they and you will be touched beyond joy, will journey to places inside and outside your hearts that will make life so much more vibrant for both of you and will give you insight and understanding of community—community as human beings who need to love, care for, and nurture each other.

The beauty of this book is that it links veterans across wars with a common redemptive thread . . . that of communion with each other and with the birds of the air. Each brings its own way of healing and recovery, soul-searching and salvation. It takes more than a village to understand that life and living, health and healing, recovery and reconciliation, love and faith are what make us human and part of that community of which John Donne so aptly wrote centuries ago, "No man is an island, entire of itself; every man is a piece of the continent, a part of the main." We heed those words simply by being present in the lives of us all.

Preface

BY JACQUELYN M. HOWARD

More than five hundred thousand U.S. troops have been wounded in recent conflicts, many of them suffering traumatic brain injuries, amputations, severe burns, and post-traumatic stress disorder (PTSD). Not all wounds from combat are visible. Twenty percent of service members returning from Iraq and Afghanistan, or three hundred thousand troops, have and will report symptoms of PTSD or major depression, according to the Wounded Warrior Project (*http://www.woundedwarriorproject.org/*, figures as of April 2010). *Wounded Warriors: A Soldier's Story of Healing through Birds* is one soldier's story about the healing and recuperative power of birds and bird watching. This story details the determined effort of one solider, Robert Vallieres, to find his "new normal" after severe internal injuries that he suffered in a vehicle equipment accident in Kuwait left him invisibly wounded and in constant pain. With little hope of functioning the way he had before he left for war, he prayed for the kind of help not found in clinics, bottles of painkillers, and behavior modification pills—and even for the comfort that was beyond what his family could offer.

One day when hope seemed out of reach, Robert mindlessly thumbed through a small local weekly newspaper, flipping the pages without reading a single word. Suddenly he noticed a small box ad for a bird-watching trip to see raptors in the mountains of New Hampshire. He read the few sentences again and felt an inexorable pull to go on this trip. He realized that the location was close by and the trip was doable: he could drive his car to the mountains and watch birds instead of feeling the pain of his disability. For the first time since his accident, he sensed that beyond suffering there might be healing. He suddenly thought of the Emily Dickinson lines

Hope is the thing with feathers
That perches in the soul,
And sings the tune without the words,
And never stops at all

This, then, is Robert's story of self-healing from crippling wounds to his back, neck, and head—wounds not always validated by those who see him as apparently whole and undamaged by the rigors of war. But he is wounded, one of the thousands of military personnel who have what are termed "invisible wounds"—traumatic brain injury (TBI) and PTSD.

Bird watching, as a therapeutic and healing modality, is unique in that it is easily accessible (birds are close by: in our backyards, in city parks, at the beach, in the mountains, and in our favorite books), requires no special equipment (just a guidebook and binoculars), can be enjoyed indoors or out, and can be done on one's own or with family members, friends, colleagues, medical staff, and others. As Robert says,

Birds saved my life. If it weren't for my connection with them, I don't know what would've happened to me. I now work with hawks and eagles through my volunteer work at the New Hampshire Audubon Center and connect with people from all walks of life. The birds and the birding community have been such a gift to me. I'm in favor of offering this kind of therapy to all incoming and recovering veterans who are in need of a safe, meditative, and calming activity that allows for participation by family members, friends, and the bird-watching public. It would've helped me greatly if there'd been such an opportunity when I was a patient at Walter Reed and especially when I out-processed to my home in rural New Hampshire. In fact, my current therapist would like to hear more about how he could use bird study in his practice where he assists wounded and other disabled vets.

As Robert's situation shows, medicine and medical interventions can do only so much. As postmobilization veterans in my office at Army National Guard Headquarters have told me, "Often, all we need is someone to just listen to us without comment, instead of trying to diagnose us or label us as casualties." I agree with them that sometimes it is not a health-care provider who can help best, but a new buddy, a volunteer, people who care and reach out with their hearts and their binoculars, offering simply to listen, to go for a walk, and . . . to watch birds.

Please consider this book a nonmedical, nonprescriptive formula that can help others like Robert, anywhere and anytime. He and I hope it spreads the word to other Wounded Warriors, veterans, and their families, reminding them that healing can happen and often lies as close as their own backyards.

Acknowledgments

We wish to express our eternal gratitude to the following people for helping us and guiding us through the monumental task of seeing this book to completion: Kate Gleason, friend, mentor, poet, and life's saving grace; Elizabeth Demers, for her belief in this project; Sam Dorrance and Ann Baker, who took the project to final publication; Carol and Andrew Vallieres, wife and son of Robert; siblings Claude, Donald, Lise, Marie, Joseph, and Roselle Vallieres; mother Yolande; World War II veteran and father Charles; Sergeant First Class Frances Hinton; Lieutenant Colonel Michael Mismash; Major Greg Arnold; Colonel Kimberly O'Keefe; Dr. Fredric Abramson, for his time and insights into the world of self-authentication; Christopher Martin and the rest of the staff of the New Hampshire Audubon Society; Larry Pelland; Maria Colbe, wildlife rehabilitator; Brett Wood, soldier, friend, and writer-to-be; Frank Orr, recruiter way back when; Al Porsche, counselor and Vietnam War veteran; Willem Lang, outdoor adventurer and storyteller; Joe Nadeau; Paul and Rhea St. Onge; Austin Hamilton; Andy Cote; Donald Cote; Lise Sanschagrin and her husband; Woodrow Purchell; Father Richard Roberge; St. John the Evangelist Catholic Church, Concord, New Hampshire; Bart Smith; Scott Owens; James O. Scott; doctors and staffs of the following: US Naval Ship *Comfort*, Walter Reed Army Medical Center, Womack Army Medical Center, Roxbury, Massachusetts, and Concord Veterans Affairs Medical Center, Concord, New Hampshire; pastor and parishioners of Faith Community Chapel, Ft. Bragg, North Carolina; and the many other medical and religious people who cared for me and my family and continue to do so. We would also like to thank Mark

Suomala, friend and fellow bird enthusiast; the Fogelmans, Susan and Wevil; Eric Masterson; Mark Vallieres; Tom Ricardi; Concord Fire and Rescue; Joni Eareckson Tada, evangelical Christian author, radio host, and founder of Joni and Friends, an organization focused on Christian ministry in the disability community; Hal Poiseau, friend and mentor; Tony Moskiewicz, Veterans Administration counselor and fellow veteran; John Howard and Kimberley Guyette; James Howard and Roxanne Streeter; Matthew Tarosky and Judith Howard Tarosky; Jean Marie and John Paul Howard, beloved parents; George Angehr, birder extraordinaire and dear friend; Lisa Barnett, mentor, confidante, colleague, and friend for life; Uncle Bob and Aunt Dee Howard; and the many contributors to Ms. Howard's first book, some of whom are quoted again in this book. We also acknowledge the many others who have supported and continue to support us in so many ways throughout this process and beyond, and we regret if in our fallibility we have forgotten you, but please know you have our eternal and everlasting thanks and gratitude.

Finally, we salute the men and women in uniform, from those on the front lines to those back home, heroes all, who serve this country well, giving of their time, their sacred honor, and sometimes their lives in the performance of their duties during peace and war. May God bless them, keep them safe, and always bring them home to those who love them.

Introduction

*In the beginning God created the heaven and the
earth. And the earth was without form, and void;
and darkness was upon the face of the deep.*
~Genesis 1:1–2

You lose things when you go to war and come back—especially when
you come back missing things like part of your brain and the whole left
ventricle of your heart. Memories are stored in both places. Not that
I've forgotten everything, but there are blanks in the memories, like
a whiteout during a snowstorm. Things are missing that you know are
there, like the shoulder of the road or the center line, but you can't see
them. You have to imagine they are there or be lucky enough to have
a passenger constantly telling you that they are, so you don't drive the
car into a ditch or worse.

My name is Robert Vallieres. I am not a Wounded Warrior. Or maybe I
am. You see, I was wounded before there was a thing called a "Wounded
Warrior." I was injured in the First Gulf War, the Persian Gulf War waged
by the UN and under President George H.W. Bush from 2 August 1990
through 28 February 1991. I'm one of the thousands of veterans with
Gulf War syndrome (GWS), that acronymic catchall for a list of ailments
considered more chronic than acute, undiagnosable.

But I don't want to be an acronym, not a GWS, TBI, PTSD, or any
other clinical term that's thrown around these days. I don't view myself
as Robert Disabled. I view myself as Robert Abled. Being labeled with
general, rather than specific, terms doesn't help me heal. Maybe some

soldiers feel better by belonging to disabled vets or Wounded Warrior organizations. They help but I feel we need to go beyond that. After all, aren't *all people* disabled in some fundamental part of their being? Aren't we all in stages of post-traumatic stress? I've even heard of people who say they have birth trauma from when they were born. So I guess we're all "post" something or other. I feel stressed every time I get up in the morning, sit behind the wheel of my truck, or go to bed at night. So, believe me, I get the "post" in post-traumatic stress, but I wish the "disorder" part of the label would go away.

Besides, I outgrew labels and diagnoses, and feeling like prey to those who categorize me as something less than whole but not yet broken into small enough pieces to ignore or put in a cage like an injured bird. Sometimes I feel like I'm surrounded by vultures that are poking, prodding, questioning me, chewing on my hapless butt, and wondering when I will relapse, collapse, weaken, and die. Then they can come up with a newer acronym, write a paper, and get known by their peers (who are hoping to do the same).

Stop the merry-go-round and just go birding; give your tired, your poor, your wounded bodies, minds, and souls to them and let the healing begin.

WOUNDED WARRIORS

1

Inglorious Injury

I am like a desert owl, like an owl among the ruins. I lie
awake; I have become like a bird alone on a roof.
~Psalms 102:6–7

Peregrine Falcons Recon at Russell Crag, White Mountains
25 May 2011; Clear, Sunny, 50°F

4:00 A.M.
In bed and alarm goes off. My mind flashes back to sirens going off, Scud missiles, and barracks. I hug my pillow close and enjoy the comfort of not being back there. I jump out of sleep, remember being awakened by the raucous voice of the drill sergeant. I'm RFO (ready for deployment). I get dressed and check my Ready, a backpack stuffed with compass, bird book, map, first aid kit, water, and food—provisions for my "deployment to falcon territory." I sling the backpack across my shoulder, grab my scope, and hurry out to the car. For a moment it feels strange to have no gun or body armor, to not be jumping into a Humvee or troop transporter but into my own car, armed only with a pair of binoculars, a birding scope, and stuff a civilian carries for a day in the mountains. I put the key in the ignition and head for Route 93 North. An hour later I reach Exit 31 and veer off the highway onto a secondary road just as the first light of day awakens the sky and earth, illuminating the forest and outlining individual mountain peaks. A sense of place and purpose infuses my heart, mind, eyes—the inexorable, primeval pull back to raw,

untamed nature fills me from the outside in. I slow the car to prolong the moment. No enemy exists here except the one within me; I fight myself to fully grasp the blessing of being here, where I stalk my prey, the mighty peregrine. My spirits soar.

5:00 A.M.

I stand at the base of the mountain where a ledge juts out over the vertical slope of granite, hanging in thin air. The sun breaks free of the horizon. I look up and see blue jays flitting near the crag where the peregrines are nesting. I watch and want to yell, "If you get too close, you'll become prey to the falcons." But I know my concern won't matter at all to the birds. Ravens are also raising their young nearby, a parent bird carrying food to a noisy brood poking their beaks out over the edge of the ungainly stick nest resting on an open ledge.

I come here to answer my call of the wild and nobody else's. But instead I fall prey to black flies that dispel any notion that wild means anything other than lack of human presence. I slap at my exposed skin, hoping to deny them their blood meal, and pray the wind picks up enough to keep them away.

As I climb to my perch under the crag where the peregrines nest, I pass an old miner's camp and keep trekking through the junglelike tangle of White Mountain National Forest, marveling at its beauty. I hear warblers singing and the nasal "whang, whang, whang" of white-breasted nuthatches and the ethereal flutes of two or three types of thrushes (wood, hermit, and, off in the distance, veery, I think). I feel centered by these mesmerizing sounds even amid the constant drone and buzz of the damn black flies. Time to pull down the sleeves of my shirt and put on more bug juice. As I spray the insect repellent all over me, I get a sharp whiff of it up my nose and . . .

. . . *I am momentarily paralyzed by the sound of biochemical and air attack sirens, Scud missiles going off. Time to strap on the protective mask, vest, helmet, and sunglasses and make my way outside into searing heat and relentless beige nothingness. My body's covered from top to bottom in the same colorless drab, damn hot and no relief. I look around me, this wasteland of hurt, of heat, of hell—my valley of death. I taste the smell of jet fuel, burned into my brain, my mouth, my nostrils, and my soul; taste it as I inhale and exhale . . .*

I shake my head, full of ache at the flashbacks and the way they swing me from here to way back there, two decades and still the "swimming in the stench of jet fuel" haunts my memory. I struggle to refocus on the birds, the winged beings that have brought me here. The birds call me back home to here and now, the invisible presence of their voices giving me rest and purpose.

7:50 A.M.

I lift myself over the edge of the crag. One of the adult peregrines zips past me and drops out of sight. Seconds later, it reappears and then swoops into an invisible split farther up the vertical rock face. Carefully I climb upward to a ledge just above the cave mine, moving with stealth . . .

. . . always with stealth, movement without disturbance, concealed without being observed. . . . My desert camo blends me into the background of sand and sun and flat foreverness—unforgiving land, colored dun, and with nowhere to hide . . .

As the difficulty of the climb increases, sweat stings my eyes. I swipe it away with the back of my hand, feel my spirit sliding out of my chest and into the forest, merging with the cool green, the soothing shade, the moldy brown, and the slippery damp. I blend into the background of shadowy greenery and dappled sun, barren outcrops and sheer rock faces. I locate the abandoned mine and wonder what was extracted from it. My objective is to remain unseen by my target, the peregrine falcon that I'm stalking. But the peregrine is not the enemy. It's my savior, my angel of mercy, my redemption from a life interrupted by a wound of war; I cry here and only God and his creatures of the earth hear me . . . no judgment, only forgiving grace. . . . Redemption.

My goal today is to confirm that a pair of falcons is here and that hatching has occurred with resultant young in the nest and to determine whether the adults are banded. I find a suitable spot where I can set up my bird scope and recon the area. The angle is extreme, but it's the best I can do. Birding is like being a soldier in war; you can only do the best you can do. As I focus, a peregrine swings into view. I let go with a silent, emphatic "Yes." I continue to track the bird through the scope, and a second bird appears—two birds, two adults! One is to my right and down the rock face about seventy-five yards, the other directly above me—male and female (the female obvious because of her large size). Later I'll try to distinguish them by malar stripes, those beautiful black facial drips that define the character of all peregrines. I swing the scope after them and I feel dizzy, my head gyrating inside itself as if the actual matter of the skull is detached from its outer protective sheath of skin and hair . . .

  . . . *everything goes blurry as my eyes slip sideways, through the haze of a truck following other trucks and kicking up dust in a long brown tail; always dust, always sun, always heat; damn waves of it that conspire to blot out what's right in front of me. My looking becomes a mirage, a trancelike staring revealing nothing. And then the horrible misstep, the lack of attention to detail, and the slamming pain of the rock-hard beam punching flesh into bone, crushing my head just short of my eye; skull moves inside skin; neck wrenches back and forth. Pain and then nothing . . . hands reach up and cradle the hurt . . . are they mine or someone else's? . . .*

I shake loose from the headache, steady myself on the barrel of the scope lightly but enough to bring myself back to being on the ledge. I squeeze my eyes shut and remember the time at Fort Bragg when I mapped bird habitat for red-cockaded woodpeckers. I was part of the 20th Engineer Brigade, 30th Engineer Battalion, 175th Engineer Company and that was my assignment. Fresh out of Fort Belvoir and cartography school . . . my mom read me the letter they sent her about how proud she should be. Back then I believed all that the army said and trusted what it did and didn't do.

Red-cockaded woodpeckers, or RCWs, are endangered birds that meant nothing to me then but mean everything to me now. Not only were they endangered birds, but they were endangering the training missions of soldiers stationed at Fort Bragg: the Eighty-Second Airborne,

Green Berets, and infantry units, which needed all the air and ground space the fort had to offer to prepare for war. Back then I had no idea how big a role birds would play in my future life, no idea of the solace I'd find among them here in these high mountains, the restorative power of wildness all around me, ripe with the healing touch of cool, fresh air, the whisper of inexorable silence and expectant birdsong. It's a place where my body feels less weighed down by gravity and more like the title of that book *The Incredible Lightness of Being*, which someone gave me once but which I didn't read. A place where God is close and there's no interference between the two of you.

I spy the peregrines again, the two of them on the wing and within my scope of view. I feel myself soar with them, released from my wounds that persist even after twenty years, even after how many surgeries, therapies, acronyms, pills, and rehabs, help that doesn't really help my invisibly crippled form that has fallen from grace, imperfect now. Who would've thought these small bodies covered in feathers would be my resurrection, restoring me to a sense of wholeness? They've given me purpose and keep me from backsliding into dark, haunted places inside me when life slices me into too many small pieces. They've saved me from the rot and deterioration that can occur in these places, where you can hurt yourself with detachment.

I go weak, and I almost drop my scope, then will myself back to the solid state of ground I stand on, refocus my mind, and move beyond the mental lapses and loss of attention to detail that are the hangers-on, symptoms of my wounds from long ago and far away. Shit happened back then, but my mind and memory are foggy. The events continue their erratic replay over and over but in fragments, staccato bursts of indefinite happenings and sequencing error, a reel-to-reel tape broken yet spinning around and around with a constant slap of the broken end. Sort of like that movie *Groundhog Day*, with its never-ending repeats, but without the romance that saves the stars from having to repeat the sameness. They don't have to deal with repetitive headaches or the feeling of being lost in space voids and black holes. But I do. I see this never-ending, cycling filmstrip of me dodging the near miss of falling back there, trying to make it turn out different in the insanity of replays with no ability to go beyond the pain. I have to live and breathe beyond it, accept that it's just part of the way I am now, walk my walk among low-slung cobwebs and hazy blurs that lessen and almost disappear only when I climb alone to these high places and search for a single pair of peregrines embedded deep within a hidden fissure. That is where truth lies—just out of view and buried inside the unseen dark of a crack in the solid rock.

I can tell these peregrines are not at last year's nest ledge but farther up the granite scree slope, near the top of the second outcrop. There the overhanging ledge secures the ravens' nest, the big, bulky pile of sticks containing the hungry brood. I wonder why the ravens built their nest so close to the peregrines' haunt. I position myself to watch, sensing the peregrines deep within the crag, there in the inner darkness . . .

. . . *I lie lifeless after the hit. Later I hear that they went into my body to fix it, their hands skillfully reconstructing my heart after an aneurysm almost stopped it. Deep within the chambers they jostled, moved, sliced, and spliced it all back together: arteries remade with Poly-Graft, an elastomer-coated Dacron vascular prosthesis—a time for attention to detail by the docs. I have a piece that I carry with me now . . . like a soft tube of shed snakeskin, pale but with no scales. But I think it was months later that I learned about the heart surgery, and I was never told the two were related—the head and the heart. War becomes timeless years afterward, and does it really matter now what happened when? Stories later remembered from the perspective of distance have a way of telling themselves, presenting their own conclusions, revealing their own truths, or not. I hurt and hurt because of injuries sustained while a soldier deployed to a war zone. It really is that simple.*

I position myself just below the ledge, like a forward scout on a recon mission, and look up so that I don't disturb the birds as they fly in and out of their hidden enclave. In contrast to the ravens with their bold and in-plain-site nest, the peregrines built their nest deep within the granite fissures, laying the eggs on the rock itself, a nest hidden from an enemy's view.

10:35 A.M.

The bees buzz the blossoms. Up here things bloom at different times than in the lower elevations—Canada lilies flowering here while the trilliums are going to seed. The call of a pileated woodpecker echoes through the forest canyon, a loud, rattling call from a prehistoric era. Winter wrens pipe their flutey rhythms. Blue jays "chay, chay," and red-eyed vireos repeat their leaftop calls of "Here I am; where are you?" in a seemingly never-ending pairing of nasal notes. I see a black-and-white warbler creeping down a hemlock trunk, vocalizing its "teetsi, teetsi, teetsi" notes, its coloring like a black-and-white candy cane.

10:55 A.M.

The pileated woodpecker calls again, "kik, kik, kikikikik, kik," a primeval sound that conjures auditory visions of Jurassic Park. I wonder if there's a nest nearby, a large hole in a dead or dying tree that holds the mom and her brood of three or four Mini-Mes. A chipmunk scurries over the dog-leaf lichen by my feet. Ants are busy nearby. As I watch them hurrying across the ground, a Bible verse from Proverbs 6 comes to mind: "Go to the ant, O sluggard; consider her ways, and be wise. Without having any chief, officer, or ruler, she prepares her bread in summer and gathers her food in harvest."

My head rolls onto my chest, and all of a sudden I'm dog tired and feel like taking a nap. I realize I've been up since 4:00 a.m., have hiked and blazed some of my own trail to get up here, and am being lulled into sleepiness by the peacefulness of where I am. "Exhaustion creep," as I call it now, is always with me, a result of my injury to head and heart, but no time for a nap now. Need to keep awake and so I focus on a bit of orange tape I tied to a nearby branch as a trail marker and watch as the breeze knocks the tape against a dead leaf, back and forth, back and forth. This is the only sound now, a crisped oak leaf, brown and crinkly, left over from last fall as it knells back and forth like the clapper in a bell, like the one encased in the bell in the steeple in the Mary Baker Eddy Church in Manchester. It keeps breaking the stillness with a barely discernible click, like the sound of a silencer being attached to a gun. A dead leaf hanging on, against all odds . . .

. . . a beam slams into my head, gouging into my skull; my spine twists as I fall. Pain but no blood; a silent and invisible rearranging of bones inside the skin. I check and all my limbs are intact—my eyes still see, my ears still hear—but something has gone terribly wrong. A pressure I can't relieve no matter which way I turn. Medics come and place me on a stretcher, locked in so my body can't move. I close my eyes . . . or was it just my buddies who picked me up and carried me in their interlocked hands and arms? . . . Imperfect memory clouds the facts but does not change the story. . . . I'm downed by friendly fire, by a damn mistake, a mishandling of the mission, and in that split second my life changed, spun out of control irrevocably . . .

10:57 A.M.

Exhaustion creep is still with me, my head droops forward, I still want a nap but tell myself, "I can do this. It's hard but I can do this. . . . Focus, focus, focus, you are on a mission." It's tough, but it's the deal now if I want to spend time wrapped in nature, alone on a mountainside, and watch these magnificent soaring machines called peregrines, winging effortlessly on currents of air that are unseen but felt, the stuff of physics and God and faith—life and breath. Bodily pain loses its hold over me when I'm with these birds. I rise, swing through the air with them—a lightness of being, a full-body experience that releases me from the physicality imposed on me by gravity and bones full of marrow. Up here, solitary and alone, where rock touches sky and trees give way to barren outcrops, I touch my scar and smile. I am the mountain carved into flesh.

Gratitude floods me. After all, I still have my eyes, ears, and limbs. I still have my sense of being, my rebuilt heart and ability to breathe . . . life's essentials. But I hurt from the inside out, in places where others cannot go, cannot understand, cannot feel and comfort, and that is why I come here—to lay bare the inside of me to God and nature and let the healing continue, let my tears roll exposed and unquestioned, while I rest on the cool green floor of the forest, looking straight up, tucked under the blue and white of heaven, birds silhouetted there against the roof of earthbound sanctity.

I look up again at the peregrines, the Blue Angels of the bird world. I am made whole by their being in my world, by the privilege of my being in their world. I give them my full attention and forget.

11:20 A.M.

. . . until a Black Hawk helicopter flies by overhead, similar to the one in which I was medevaced . . . the whup-whup of the propellers, a raucous, raking sound that unnerves my body, vibrates right through it, even way up here, miles and so much time away from back then, when . . .

. . . *I'm helped into the gaping maw of the medical evacuation helicopter; an air force medic team; head and heart pained, stiff, short of breath and with a nerve-maiming headache; bile, thick and sour, pushes up from my gut to form at the back of my throat but it is too dry to heave it up—saliva missing. Shoved in, anchored down, and then up, up, and away . . . I'm flying; lose and regain consciousness for brief moments; leaving the field of battle and I can remember only the name of the mission, Imminent Thunder. . . . I land on the deck of the U.S. Navy ship* Comfort, *touch the hand of one of the airmen, mumble thanks for bringing me here, maybe saving my life; my lips crack open and I taste blood and start speaking again, but he turns and walks away, my guardian angel, drifts off onto the deck of a floating hospital anchored in the Mediterranean, ocean water as blue as sky and wet as the desert sand is dun and dry . . . life and war are full of contrasts that sharpen the thin slip of awareness; death is only a breath or a heartbeat away from life . . .*

I squeeze my forehead between the flats of my palms. Sometimes I don't know what's real and what's not. Time's a sliding scale that works against perfect memory. So, was there a Black Hawk buzzing the air way up here where I'm watching peregrines? Is that the chopper I was taken away in over in the Saudi desert? Then I hear the falcon chicks begging for food. Sounds like two of them. . . . I shake and draw my mind and memory back to the ledge and to the present. I know that watching these young peregrines mate, unedited and unscripted, is better than any other therapy prescribed by any number of doctors who have worked on me.

This is my antidote to all that came before, a real and unconditional dose of nature where life and death have no conscience and no remedy; it's distilled to its essence and that is survival with no consequences.

11:30 A.M.

The male peregrine flies out from within the crag. Ten minutes later it flies back, prey clutched in its claws—a small animal, maybe a bird, I can't tell. The female flies out from her hidden lair. The male offers her the prey and she grasps it in her talons, all done in midair. Reminds me of a KC10 refueling a jet in midflight. I saw that once and was in awe. She quickly disappears into the crevice in the ledge. As suddenly as she disappeared, she reappears. The young must be hungry.

. . . I am hooked up and the intravenous fluid pumps into me, refuels my body; the nurses, both male and female, tend me, all in white; clean, young-looking faces; they constantly appear and disappear . . . slide a table alongside the bed, offer food but I'm not hungry . . . make me swallow pills, rearrange my pillow, smile, grab my wrist, count my pulse in beats per minute; smell antiseptic and slightly pharmaceutical . . .

11:50 A.M.

Now both parents are outside the nest. I determine that they are feeding two, maybe three, hatchlings. Today's mission accomplished and objectives met—pair confirmed, young present in nest, adults not banded.

. . . I never met my objective that day, never completed the mission, a simple one, offloading construction material—beams. Did I fail the mission or did the mission fail me? Could I have done anything differently? Not deployed? Gotten a medical exemption for a bad heart? Doc said no time to file . . . ready and confirmed to fight the good fight—expendable . . . and now I deal with anger, frustration, pain, betrayals, and the tag of disabled. Wish I were a peregrine feeding two young in a nest high up in the White Mountains of New Hampshire, unseen and inaccessible, not known to exist but just existing . . .

12:10 P.M.

. . . but I am here and this is my life, for better or worse or somewhere in between. Comfort, clarity, the elusiveness of trying to be myself, not someone else, not a diagnosis, a bottle of painkillers, a remnant of humanity, a casualty, a being perfectly formed outwardly but with internal damage. How do I be me? No one else can wear my skin, feel my sensations, know what I seek way up here . . . words are weak substitutes for conveying this duality.

Before heading back down the mountain, I flip my journal to its inside cover, where I've pasted a quote from Henry David Thoreau, and I read it aloud:

> I went to the woods because I wished to live deliberately, to front only the essential facts of life, and see if I could learn what it had to teach, and not, when I came to die, discover that I had not lived. I did not wish to live what is not life, living is so dear; nor did I wish to practice resignation, unless it was quite necessary. I wanted to live deep and suck out all the marrow of life, to live so sturdily and Spartan-like as to put to rout all that was not life, to cut a broad swath and shave close, to drive life into a corner, and reduce it to its lowest terms, and if it proved to be mean, why then to get the whole genuine meanness of it, and publish its meanness to the world; or if it were sublime, to know it by experience, and be able to give a true account of it in my next excursion. For most men, it appears to me, are in strange uncertainty about it, whether it is of the devil or of God.

Thoreau helps me at least to understand myself better. I get it, what he said so many decades ago. I understand it literally, for my life was almost lost, to a hot desert, in a very far-off place, where I didn't hear so clearly the drumbeat of my own heart. I was a young soldier, deployed to a war zone, and then my head crumpled and my heart burst, stopped beating, was torn open and rebuilt to start again. My life at the brink of death was not sublime. I did not need to imagine losing it, for I did and, by the grace of God, was given another chance.

The mountain has been good to me today, and the peregrines are recorded in my journal. I now am satisfied and make my journey back down to where rock gives way to woods and finally to flat land where my car is waiting. Success is measured in many ways, and today has been a success.

I wonder why doctors don't give out prescriptions for reading Thoreau or taking up bird watching. Reading Thoreau's words could do more to heal people than all the remedies in the medical toolbox, and watching birds fly and cut the air high above the shallow, sculpted notch below a remote wilderness in northern New Hampshire just could be the antidote, a homegrown remedy and drug-free cure with no warning labels attached.

2

Invisible Wounds

Inside the soul,
right in the very middle of it,
there's a bird standing on one foot.
This is the soul bird.
It feels everything we feel.
~Michal Snunit, *The Soul Bird*

Peregrine Falcons Recon at Russell Crag
7 May 2011; High Overcast, Breezy, 60s F

5:20 A.M.
Tripoli Road; right side of the road near speed limit sign. I pull over and park the car, roll down the window and listen. I hear a peregrine calling, six times with "whine" call notes . . .

... *Rolling down the window of the jeep I look for signs of red-cockaded woodpecker holes in the loblolly pines; note a hole in a tree on the right side of the road near speed limit sign; pull over and hear a faint hammering five or maybe six times. I note coordinates on the base map of Fort Bragg resting in my lap. Winds calm, high overcast, but hot as hell even in early morning. Humidity lives down here like it's the devil's breath. It breathes all over you until you're wet and soggy and chaffing—inside your skin and outside your skin . . .*

5:30 A.M.
Just found a large stick nest supported between white birches . . .

. . . Found it! Large hole fifteen feet up in tree about fifty feet in from tank trail; note large amount of whitish sap oozing down trunk. I've been told that this means an active nesting cavity but could also be a false positive. Damn woodpeckers are pretty clever with their fake nest holes and shit like that.

5:34 A.M.

Again hear three-note whine; nest is covered in whitewash; raucous call once; four-note whine, then three-note whine. Only one bird calling. Need to listen and watch . . . need to know if there's a pair or just a single bird?

5:37 A.M.

Two more cry notes; peregrine cry persistent—seven-note whine, five-note whine, eight-note whine, four-note, three-note, four-note, cries a whining call, four-note, two-note, five-note, three-note.

5:49 A.M.

Single peregrine still calling . . . mournful and echoing off the hollows of the cliff face.

6:00 A.M.

Six-note, three-note, six-note whine calls, followed by a series of a single-cry notes, three-note, and then six-note whines.

6:05 A.M.

More of the same. Multiple whine notes with an occasional cry note . . . then a second, far-distant response! Pair of peregrines calling. I look all around, first with just my eyes and then with binos to the ready but cannot locate the other bird. It calls again and I confirm the pair . . .

. . . I stop and look around me. Everything looks the same in a loblolly forest—sandy ground, dry and pungent with the smell of fallen and decaying needles, a clumpy grass called wire grass. We don't have any of this up north, but pines are pines and this forest has a similar, almost familiar smell to it, sort of like a white pine forest up north. Almost 0630 and heading back soon, mission accomplished. These woodpeckers come out of their holes before

sunrise and then come back just at dusk, so no use scouting around for drill holes during the day. Pack it in at 0700 and head for chow.

6:25 A.M.

All is quiet; why? Did I blank out and miss something essential happening? Did I have a minor seizure or just a pause in consciousness, even though I am still standing and my eyes are open? This stuff happens to me, and no one can tell me why, like I fall asleep for a minute or two and miss what's right in front of me. Damn, what did I miss?

. . . I crumple to the ground, grabbing my head in pain so intense I see bolts of white light screaming behind my eyes. Vomit crawls up the back of my throat. God, don't let me piss in my pants. . . . I can't stop the tears. . . . What the hell just happened?

Still no peregrines calling; only silence and my missing it, whatever it was. Was it a predator that I didn't see, a raven's shadow overhead that silenced the peregrine, or something else? I was watching and scanning the area around the nest with my scope but missed it, that's all. Could have been a raven? I didn't see anything flying but I wouldn't during my blank out; shit, this happens sometimes. I just lose it to the moment, to the instant that passes quickly, in the blink of an eye or the intake of a breath, lose what's right in front of me. It's like there's a void, a vacuum, a black hole, a wrinkle in my space-time continuum, and there I am, missing in action, again.

I go over every detail again but still can't ever go back and pick up the missing time, the hole in the sequence of events. But wait, a raven isn't a predator of adult peregrines. But is it a nest predator of young peregrines still unable to fly? Or would a raven try to reclaim the nest? Only if the peregrine were using a raven's nest from the previous nesting season. Confusion often is my companion, works on me like spaghetti winding and unwinding on a fork, sometimes you get it right and sometimes it just all unravels on you, leaving you wondering what went missing in the process. I wait and watch intently. I hear a raven call far off in the distance. I'm winding and unwinding what happened, I have only questions with no answers. I'm waiting on the peregrines to start the time again so I can go from there . . .

6:58 A.M.
Silence so pure I can hear blood rushing inside the veins of my ears. No peregrines calling. Was I looking at the correct spot? I'm not exactly sure what happened here, but I just missed it. I'd been looking straight out at the ledge but I lost it, dropped the ball, just like before when I missed the beam that tore at my head. The moment that something happened, I was MIA. I wasn't paying attention, but what if it's not your fault but someone else's? That's why I'm still here, to try to understand if the peregrines were calling for help and I didn't even know it. Maybe not their fault but the fault of an unseen predator or an accident? Or was it me that caused the peregrines to stop calling, to go into hiding or die?

7:00 A.M.
Still in place. Three ducks fly by, heading west. Was the falcon somewhere near the nest when it stopped calling, moving, being visible to me? Is there a nest? I just assumed but now really don't know. Dark clouds descend upon me at Russell Craig . . .

. . . I fall to my knees, cradle my head, waft in and out of semiconsciousness. Darkness blackens me; my eyes screw shut, then splay open, but I see only dark that makes me cold like air conditioning on high, chilling the inside of my skin, that layer where nerves are right at the surface; my eyes dry out, lids scrape against pupils; hurts like hell; I gulp for air and taste a lack of moisture, just parched dryness; my eyes are stuck open and I see too much light; can't blink, too painful. I'm writhing in pain in the desert sand and cannot close my eyes . . .

7:12 A.M.
I decide to move around the cliff side and find a better clearing to see the ledge. I hear a motorcyclist whiz by way down below on the road.

7:46 A.M.

I hear cries and look up at a clearing to the right of where I was originally sitting. I see falcons, a pair of them, swooping and soaring in and out of cloud and sun . . .

. . . guys in my unit are shouting and moving above me, calling for help. I hope someone hears them, pays attention to them, someone who can help and knows what to do. I can't move, lying still and corpse-like on the Saudi desert grittiness where above you is nothing but sky without hope of shade . . .

7:48 A.M.

I look up, down, in front, and behind me and—voila—I can see the nest! I wonder how I missed it before. Peregrines and their nest are all accounted for. Birds are alive and well. And better still, one of the adults has prey grasped tightly in its talons. I watch as the one adult approaches the other and a prey exchange occurs—one offers prey, a dead meal offering, and the other takes it, a sure sign of mating and courtship. After this ritual, they fly away in opposite directions from each other. Then the one with the prey circles and lands on a pale, whitish rock face, a slight jutting out of a ledge that offers a perfectly protected perch. She is the larger of the two and so I identify her as the female. She begins to pick and pull at the bloodied morsel tightly held between the talons of her left foot, a love offering from her mate, the much smaller male. I'm now relieved that my thinking the peregrines were dead was unfounded. They have risen, and I think of God speaking to those with patience—James 1:2-4: "My brethren, count it all joy when you fall into various trials, knowing that the testing of your faith produces patience. But let patience have its perfect work, that you may be perfect and complete, lacking nothing."

7:50 A.M.

I'm back at the base of the mountain. My day is now done, and all is well. Not sure where the falcon who gave his mate the prey went, but maybe to where the nest is. I'm at peace that both falcons are present, alive and well! I reach for my keys deep in my pants pocket, pull them out, and start the car. As I pull away from the shoulder, I know that this pair of peregrines is going to be okay . . .

. . . Am I going to be okay? I reach for my buddy's arm and hold on. And then the sun goes out in the midday desert and the last thing I remember is slamming into hot sand and grit . . .

I'm wounded still, even after two decades, wounded more on the inside. Sometimes, but only sometimes, I wish my wounds were more obvious and easier to see. That way people wouldn't keep looking at me funny when they ask me about what I do for work. I can't work like others work. The wounds prevent that, the exhaustion, killer fatigue, pounding, spike-driven headaches, seizures, inability to use technology the way it ought to be used, forgetfulness, nausea, and bouts of depression. Doc calls it PTSD, or post-traumatic stress disorder. So I carry the wounds under cover of skin and clothes. Wounds you can't see, wounds from a noncombat mission. Two strikes against me. Now I add embarrassment to the list of wounds, but that's more a wound of having my integrity questioned by others than an actual wound that matters to my body. But it still hurts, makes me cringe and get angry. People mean well, I suppose, but are ignorant. They like to give voice to their ignorance and no one questions what real dopes they are when it comes to having even the slightest idea of what type of injuries I've sustained. I've learned that wounds come in many forms and those sustained in a war have to be treated as equally valid and named as war wounds, whether glorious or inglorious. But it's hard having to convince others who don't want to believe you. Perhaps the unbelievers are the wounded, and we wounded are the okay ones. I need to think on that. Besides, glorious war wounds usually end your life or leave bits and pieces of you back at the scene. That's what the dopes want to see and hear about, not about me, the walking wounded with invisible scars that won't heal.

Peregrine Falcon Observations, Frankenstein Cliff
6 June 2007; Variably Cloudy, 59°F

9:35 A.M.

Driving along listening to Fleetwood Mac's "Dragonfly" followed by Bon Jovi's "The Distance" on the radio. At Exit 18 I note a loose bundle of roses and carnations with daisies sprinkled in, red as blood and white as hope that springs eternal, laying explosed at the base of a big pine tree—a makeshift memorial where someone died. Daisies bloom in May, not in April, and roses only deep into summertime in New Hampshire. But they bloom whenever you want them to, through music, on the radio, in your mind.

10:18 A.M.

I veer off the highway and head for Cannon Mountain. Been told there's a bear hanging out on the ski slope. And sure enough, there it is!

10:23 A.M.

I crank up the volume on a French radio station that I can get way up here in north central New Hampshire.

10:25 A.M.

Je vais les montagnes pour chercher des falcons, je suis heureux. . . I go to the mountains to see falcons, I am happy. It is good to still remember my first language and use it, good that I can still remember it, with all that has happened since I was made to learn English when I entered high school, when the New Hampshire government changed the rules and banned all teachers from teaching us in French.

10:33 A.M.

Twin Mountain turnoff . . .

. . . turned and puked my guts out; told the doc my head was not right, not right enough for me to go back on duty; why didn't he listen to me; nausea, headaches, gut ache . . . edge of being sick and the damn siren blasting

its warning. . . . Scud attack imminent and I stumble for cover . . . je suis malade, je suis damn malade. . . *and grab my gas mask . . .*

10:52 A.M.
Arrive Frankenstein Cliff—54°F; immediately observe prey exchange in midair out in front of cliff face: one peregrine flies from the right side of cliff to meet the other peregrine coming from the left side and prey exchange occurs in midair. I lose sight of them, but then I pick up one that I follow as it flies into a triangular rock ledge just above where a previous year's stick nest was located; the triangular feature is where the nest is and is near the top of the cliff face. Winds are moderate to heavy and it's cool. My scope shakes and some heat waves distort the view in my scope. I'm watching only this section of the cliff, which is where I observed activity during my last visit, so I think this is where the nest is. There's no way to determine which peregrine (male or female) had the prey.

. . . *Frankenstein Cliff—rugged, jagged, sinewy scar that is etched across the face of underlying smooth granite, like the one now on my chest, rough-stitched cross-hatching running across and up and down the broad plank of my upper body. I smile, thinking of this analogy imprinted not only in my eye-scape but across my chest, thanks to the surgeon who cut me open with his knife and then stitched me back together . . . the topography of the peregrine's aerie etched forever on me . . .*

12:35 P.M.
Observe a small mammal—chipmunk or red squirrel—scurrying across the ledge then quickly running away. My eyes water from the wind. I want to hike into the shelter of the cliff.

1:09 P.M.
Peregrine flies into triangular area, lands, and pauses on ledge. Other peregrine gets up and flies out. The smaller male is the one coming out of the nesting area. The larger female that flew in pauses; male flies off and female walks into crevice and out of sight.

2:08 P.M.
I am privileged to be here, privileged to watch these birds of the air and of the earth. I thank God for instilling this goodness in my life. In celebration I offer you this, my beloved birds, my teachers, healers, killers of the pain—the memories that haunt my inner life. Here's to you, my nesting pair! Pair confirmed! Nesting confirmed! And thank thee, Lord, for the gift of today; thank thee, Lord, for the birds of prey; thank thee, Lord, for the gift of today; thank thee, Lord, for the birds to which I pray. Today I thank thee, Lord.

4:10 P.M.
Time to go. I pack out and hump back down the mountainside.

6:15 P.M.
At truck and it's 51°F with stiff and gusty winds.

6:25 P.M.
Pull out for home and tune into *Blackberry Time* on the radio—a good song by Judd Kerrywell but didn't catch the name. Farther on down the road, I crank up French radio station 102.7 and listen to "Le corbeau chanson" (Raven song) and "Il y a vie" (There is life).

8:04 P.M.
Back home. Once inside I finish writing in my notebook the following entry: "Good day but cold. Numb fingers. Saw bear feeding at Cannon Ski Area; saw five ravens dancing in the winds above Mt. Webster. Doing my share for nature's sake. Tallied 193 miles round-trip." I give a quiet moment of thanks and pencil down one of the Bible's most memorable and healing quotes from Matthew 17:20: "I say to you, if you have faith the size of a mustard seed, you will say to this mountain, 'Move from here to there,' and it will move. Nothing will be impossible for you." Today is the day I climbed and felt my burden shift, if only for this time I spent closer to heaven in the realm of the peregrines, alone and yet not alone, a place where I'm tucked away from judgments, where all is full of air and sky and invisible movements. Why is it possible for

some to believe in the invisible movements of air and clouds and not the invisible wounds, the hurt, I carry inside? Do we doubt most when it is our own species and yet believe more when it isn't?

Peregrine Falcon Breeding Survey at Russell Crag
12 May 2011; Warm, Partly Sunny, 60s F

Peregrine falcon breeding sites: Abenaki Mountain, Devil's Slide, Mt. Willard, Eaglet Spire, Sugarloaf Mountain, Russell Crag, Rattlesnake Mountain, Square Ledge, Painted Walls, Cathedral Ledge, Frankenstein Cliff, Holt's Ledge, Littleton, Manchester . . . names ranging from descriptive, sublime, and animated to mundane. Today I'm at my favorite place, Russell Crag, and spring migration is in full swing.

5:30 A.M.
I come back here year after year, as does the pair of peregrines. No matter how many times I return, I discover new things about the birds, the habitat, myself. I wander back, let the gears of time slide against the inevitability of things forgotten, until they're found again—a pathway to a memory housed inside a damaged mind—figure eights sketched across the ice on a placid, frozen lake; a hand held while I said "I do"; wet socks drying, sizzling, and seizing on the iron radiator; me, a recruit, leaving for basic training; me and how I got here from there, back to New Hampshire, humping up the White Mountains, watching birds, birds watching over me . . .

. . . I'm dying. I'm cold in a hot place and see angels hovering above me. But then I'm scratching frost from the inside pane of the window in the upstairs bedroom that I share with my three brothers. Not unusual in January in Berlin, New Hampshire, the town I live in. I lived here twice in my life, from birth through sixth grade and then again in ninth grade. In between the family grew, spilt up, and I with them. Parents divorced, I was shipped to Arizona for two years to live with my oldest brother and then back to New Hampshire to live with my older sister in Berlin and then to Manchester to finish my last three years of high school living with my mom. I remember, my senior year,

yelling downstairs to my mother and asking if the mail had come. I'm wait-
ing for my army enlistment letter. I look forward to becoming a soldier; just
six months till I graduate. I've already decided that I'm going to be a career
soldier and see the world and get an education. Life will be good once I join
the army. Two weeks later I get my enlistment letter. I'm in . . . but deferred
for one year. That's okay. But suddenly I'm dying so far from home. Mom,
I love you, I hear a strange yet familiar voice, mine, say. Someone shouts,
"Hey, we're not your mom; hey, kid, give me a sign you can see my fingers
in front of your face." Stuff's oozing out of the back of my throat. His voice
kills my voice, and then puke from my mouth lands in his lap . . .

5:38 A.M.

I hear them, a pair greeting each other. I see one of them carrying food
and disappearing behind the left cliff face. I assume he's the male bringing food to the female, who should be sitting on eggs by now. I hear their
rapid, chirpy sound of greeting and then see him swoop up and away
over the far ridge . . .

    . . . The medics move in; I feel a thumb lift my stiff and dry eyelids up
even farther into their sockets. I wince, feel the salty wet roll down my face.
They lift me in a one-two-three-lift exercise. I'm deadweight as they hoist
me up and plop me down, strapping me tight to the frame and carrying me.
I hear words of encouragement but can't speak. Eyes, mouths, voices hover
just above me. A hand touches my shoulder, my arm. Where am I? Damn,
it's hot, as hot here as it is cold in January in New Hampshire. I try to move
my caked mouth but croak out a sound not human. Someone with a needle
tells me to shut the fuck up and lie still . . .

7:48 A.M.

Sun just starting to poke above treetops. Beautiful in the New Hampshire north woods in spring. Forest shadows come alive with all sorts
of birdsong. Migration is in full swing. In a clearing I spy the peregrine
cutting the air with scythe-like precision, wings unifying body and soul,
banking, diving, disappearing, sparring with the invisible enemies of
air, wind, and sky . . . ancient scimitars. I like the word *scimitar*, a curved
blade of medieval times . . .

. . . the chopper swirls upward from the ground as gracefully as a ballet dancer, swirls upward and blows the sand in all directions. The sky is blaring bright, severely white-hot bright. I raise my arm to shield my eyes. Watch as those on the ground become small dots and then disappear. I think of angels lifting me up but not quite to heaven, but this is the place where angels linger, perform miracles, the place where they bore our Lord to heaven after he died and resurrected. One last look at the ground far below before nausea and headache take over . . . war is a hellish place with such history of compassion and contempt. We either survive untouched or we bear the scars of our conflict . . .

What I learned from the battlefield is this: not everyone gets wounded in a way that validates their presence in the war. I was embarrassed to talk about my wound and how crippling it was to me because my head wasn't almost blown away by the enemy. Instead it was almost sheared off my shoulders by a fellow soldier, a known person, in my command. I was not out in front, kicking down doors, or on the roadside checking IDs, or pulling the trigger on known targets, or even in a line of transporters getting blown up by a roadside bomb. My head was punched in due to "friendly fire," so to speak. My still-alive body was messed up due to a fucking mistake made by an over excited first lieutenant not having his shit together enough to know how to unload a truck, hand off supplies, and look where he is putting things. But then the heart acted up, an old recurring ailment that the army knew all about before deployment. Sometimes I wonder if evacuation in a body bag would have been better—getting the pain and suffering over with in an instant, instead of dragging life out trying to figure out why. At least in that case there's a legitimate story to be told by those left alive after you. Now it's constant explaining and facing the look on others' faces when they see you whole and yet you are all crumbled up inside, damaged, discharged, disabled, and—worse—disbelieved.

3

Bands

Consider birdsong or bird migration. Whatever leads us to think we're the only beings capable of creating a symphony or able to commit to a single mate for life, risking everything to return to our distant place of birth? Why would we be the only ones to devote our lives to something larger than ourselves?
~Alan Tennant, "Penguins in Love"

Power Line Tower Site, Manchester
7 December 2009; Cloudy, Cool, Rainy, Low 30s F

11:48 A.M.
I pull in, park car, set up scope, and scan with binoculars. Stop and note silhouette of what appears to be a peregrine atop the middle power line tower.

12:00 P.M.
Point scope at silhouette and focus in on adult peregrine perched on middle power line tower. I jot down a few notes and take another look and see two adult peregrines flying north to south out beyond the perched peregrine on the tower. The two hug close to the horizon line, and I lose them to the flat light and low clouds—gone in sixty seconds, so to speak. I refocus on the perched peregrine; it now has turned and faces south instead of north. Seeing these birds makes the rain and clouds disappear for me, clears my brain and livens my senses, orders my disordered-ness, forcing me to focus on details—of the birds, weather, temperature,

location, winds, direction—and write them all down. I soar with these birds. Weightlessness takes over, and I am lost to the feathers around the face, the speckles on the breast, the piercing dark eyes that do not vary with age, the power of their wings, body unfettered and entire—no pain or sorrow, no sadness, anger, depression, aloneness, remorse, regret, what ifs—just one with the air and the need to survive; peregrines, flying inside my skin and outside of theirs. I am the air they use, the food they eat, the perch they grasp, the talons that kill, the beak that tears, the mate they seek and the nest they make, the thermals they seek, the migration route home; nothing to justify, nothing to know except hunger in the belly and the search for food. Winter is fast approaching, and I wonder when these peregrines will leave and fly south: before the snow flies or as it flies? They'll fly south, not by knowing and not by thinking about it . . .

. . . the medical evacuation helicopter spins its blades near where I am standing by for boarding, scuffing up dust and debris; a dry sear, scalding, dust whirled up from a vast nothingness of gritty sand. Blinding brightness shuts my eyes. I walk over and board, enjoy the sensation of the lifting up of my body under mechanical power . . .

Peregrines or chopper? Saudi or New Hampshire? Lifted up or sitting still? Displacement is what the doctors call it . . .

12:30 P.M.

New bird lands near original perched peregrine on middle power line tower and settles to its right. It's another adult peregrine, a female most likely because she's comparatively larger than the other one. She's banded on her left leg, but I can't read it. Yes, I confirm this is a female bird by comparing its size to the other bird perched nearby. He's notably smaller overall.

. . . choppers aren't the only "birds" in the desert that drop directly out of the sky. What about the Holy Spirit—the breath of God—come in for a landing on the heads of the apostles in the form of a white dove? That happened over here somewhere after Jesus left for heaven, taken up by God with the promise he would not leave them alone . . .

12:54 P.M.

Je crois en esprit saint, seigneur et donateur de la vie, qui procède à partir du père et du fils. Avec le père et le fils il est adoré et a amélioré. Il a parlé par les prophètes—I believe in the Holy Spirit, the Lord and giver of life, who proceeds from the Father and the Son. With the Father and the Son he is worshipped and glorified. He has spoken through the prophets.

I believe peregrines are made of the stuff of the Holy Spirit, and they have spoken to me through the wind that whispers and roars and sometimes whistles way up here; the sound of the breath of life emitted by the peregrines as they greet each other—that happy, high-pitched chatter, sometimes almost a rapid clicking suppressed by air and caught on the high note, syncopated, a sound uttered on air intake instead of air outtake, pressed inward instead of pushed outward; a sound like dying in the desert in a far-off place where sucking in life uttered a hope of life, and letting it out signaled a giving up.

1:00 P.M.

Female is more sooty in plumage, chest and belly dingy white to grayish; definitely one-quarter to one-third larger. The smaller male bird perched nearby is much darker plumaged and very white in the chest and belly . . .

. . . *nurses hover, all white, some larger, some smaller. "Robert, can you hear me?" a sweet voice whispers close to my face. "You're on the navy hospital ship* Comfort. *Can you hear me, see me? Don't speak now. Rest . . ."*

1:10 P.M.

Thirty robins fly south about sixty feet overhead. They add a slight streak of color against a colorless sky, breasts all rusty orange. Map skills come in handy; I can even gauge vertical distance against a limitless space. Distance is a funny business—it can be virtual or it can be real. It can be spatial or it can be temporal—or imaginary, as you can be close to someone physically but a million miles away from them on every other level. I can be sixty feet from a flock of fleeing robins yet so distant from them in capabilities that I can never reach them . . .

. . . Even when I was only ten feet away from a flying solid mass, I couldn't see it coming, couldn't reach out and stop it, couldn't hold a hand up to push it away before it hit me in the head. Distance plays into the head game of "what if." What if I'd stepped one foot to the right or one foot to the left? What if I'd hit the ground so that the beam passed over me? What if I'd been a million miles away and not deployed at that place and at that time? This mind game leaves me exhausted and self-pitying sometimes. But there's never any going backward, except in the mind, where games play out in a multiplex of scenarios that can never change the ending . . . only writers can do that and only in fiction.

1:12 P.M.
Female peregrine scratches head. I can see band clearly on left leg and record number and color sequence—black over green, 02 over Z.

1:15 P.M.
Male turns around and faces north. He suddenly takes off and flies north and comes circling back, perching almost in the same spot. Ah, I see he's banded, too. A black over green combination with 6 over 7.

1:25 P.M.
The female stretches her legs, preens, and shows me her band again.

1:27 P.M.
Female vocalizes.

1:39 P.M.
Female preens.

1:45 P.M.
Female flies off and disappears under nearby bridge. Male follows. Each makes two sorties after prey. She returns and perches, no prey. Then he returns to perch with no prey. I give this pair a name—the Queen City pair, after Manchester, the Queen City of New Hampshire.

1:50 P.M.

Fifty or so crows cackling and cawing; I cock my ear, listen, and hear a lone bald eagle scream its high-intensity note overhead, more like a tiny baby trying out its vocal chords for the first time than a robust call from a very large bird of prey and the symbol of our nation. It soars low and fast over the far horizon and then dips below my field of sight.

2:30 P.M.

Inside my vehicle now, watching the peregrines; too cold and wet outside. Female preens, and then male preens. Problem with being inside the vehicle is that I can no longer detect vocalizations, but time's running out for today. Observations today include: (1) four peregrines sighted: the male and the female that perched near him on the middle power line tower and the two observed flying that disappeared over the horizon; (2) the perched male and female appear to be a pair—one is a female and one is a male, as determined by size; both banded and I was able to record colors and numbers of each band; (3) they are adults, as determined by coloration; (4) they hunted in flight; one flight together but unsuccessful in terms of catching prey; (5) bald eagle was nearby and vocalizing; and (6) the pair of peregrines seems healthy in appearance.

   . . . *eyelid lifted, bright light pointed into eyeball, dilates pupils; eyeball squints, squirms around, tries to close itself but can't. Body stiff, mouth cracked and dry, lips stuck together like when you lick a cold ice cube on a hot day and your lips freeze onto the ice until you stick your mouth under a running faucet to free them up. Wedding band's missing . . . my band missing. Unbanded. Why? Where?*

Brady Sullivan Tower, 1750 North Elm Street, Manchester
3 May 2010; Warm, Partly Cloudy, Dry, 60s F

10:30 A.M.

Adult peregrine lands on perch near nest box.

10:35 A.M.

Peregrine looks in the nest box intently.

10:38 A.M.

Hops on ledge and goes into the nest box.

10:39 A.M.

Other adult peregrine lands atop left corner of the roof and has prey in talons.

10:40 A.M.

Plucking of prey occurring. I want to somehow capture the raw energy of this moment, the killing and the eating, the fundamentalness of life where we each have to kill to sustain our own life. Something must always be sacrificed for the other to survive. More than an emotion, this essential nature of the existence of things pervades everything, even in war, or most especially in war, where the individual is killed and consumed, used up, to keep alive the ideal, the purpose, the living and breathing war machine of human beings acting as both predator and prey. A painful mind I have sometimes, and I'm not even sure if what I think or write down makes any sense. Spaghetti prose, I call it.

10:50 A.M.

When I compare old photos I took when I started watching here at this building with new photos, I note that there weren't as many communications antennas as there are now. These make a flight hazard for the falcons.

11:03 A.M.

One of the peregrines flies out and back and lands on an antenna tower—maybe a hazard but also a perch, so there's a positive aspect to having the antennas.

11:05 A.M.

I can read the band on the adult male (smaller of the two falcons): black over green and 6 over 7.

11:25 A.M.

Peregrine male flies away and I lose sight of him. I suspect he's on what is called a hunt flight—searching for prey.

11:26 A.M.

Adult flies out of nest box, makes two aerial circles over the building, and comes back to nest box. It's a banded female; now she goes into the nest box.

11:30 A.M.

Female flies out of the nest box. This is an indication that she's not incubating eggs but may have hatchlings inside.

11:31 A.M.

Male flies by and female goes out to meet him and chirps twice. She flies back to perch on nest box . . .

. . . *I wake up and feel a hand on my forehead. Everything's small, crowded, and loud. I open my mouth to speak and puke all over myself. "Why can't I move? What's happening? Where am I? Fort Leonard Wood?" "No," a booming voice says. Someone connected to it hovers and sticks a needle in my arm. "You've been wounded. You're in Saudi Arabia, hold still." . . . don't talk . . . chopper on the way . . . swirling dust and noise . . . hoisted in and . . .*

11:32 A.M.

Male brings prey to female—prey exchange. He chirps six times; she responds with two chirps, takes prey from him, and goes to the north side of the building, out of sight, to pluck prey. Male goes to top left of the building.

11:34 A.M.

She reappears, perches momentarily outside nest box, chirps once, and enters nest box with prey. Adult male still perched on left top of building . . .

. . . *I hear the voice of Carol, my wife. Bright lights, clean sheets, hushed sounds. I'm lying in a bed, hospital of some sort. I'm captured prey to someone else's care. She is perched on the bed, hovering over me . . . adult male, adult female, banded . . .*

11:35 A.M.

All seems to be going well at this nest site—confirmed pair; confirmed hatch, as female entered nest box with prey.

. . . we are a confirmed pair. She hovers and I lose sight of her, can't keep my eyes open . . .

Fall Hawk Watch, Mary Baker Eddy Church Site, Manchester

5 October 2009; Clear, Cool, Low 50s F

8:00 A.M.

I stop by the local bagel shop before going to peregrine site. I'm doing a hawk watch, but the peregrines for me seem to fall outside that category, or actually they fall inside it but expand it outward . . .

. . . like the aneurysm did to my heart, not outside my heart but inside my heart—expanding the vessel from inside out . . . precision extraction and reconstruction; giving my life back to the world, me, my family—my angels of mercy with gifts from God above . . .

Peregrines are the upwardly mobile, high-flying, precision jet-fighter pilots of the avian world . . . Blue Angels!

8:10 A.M.

I pull car into parking garage, get scope out of backseat, set up to watch hawks. Immediately spot raptor flying, ID it as peregrine. It has a band on left leg—black over green. Bird perches on steeple.

8:30 A.M.

Peregrine flies off.

8:32 A.M.

I decide to get in my car and drive in the direction of peregrine. I stop at state hospital and get out, look up and identify a Cooper's hawk, hunting pigeons in the brightness.

. . . hospitals always nauseated me but now offer me only comfort, clean sheets, and someone taking my pulse to see if I'm alive or dead. Nurses jostle

me and put me in a wheelchair. I dangle forward. They strap me in and wheel me off to get some x-rays. I'm too weak and tired to protest, to ask for a glass of water, to go to the bathroom. And the whole crazy scene of my being sent to Portsmouth, Virginia, instead of Walter Reed in Washington DC, a mix-up because I was an army casualty, transported from theater by the air force medevac chopper to U.S. Navy hospital ship Comfort, *then to Germany, then to Portsmouth. Army and navy got me all mixed up, and no one would listen to me. So I was taken to a hospital that wouldn't help me, admit me, or transfer me for weeks. My wife was crazy worried and couldn't find me. She was told to show up at Walter Reed. She drove all night to find me MIA. All night we were within a few hours of each other, but we kept better track of each other when we were separated by almost half a world . . . and so did the army, I think.*

8:50 A.M.

I drive back to church, wait and watch . . .

. . . *Carol and I married in a Catholic church on Cape Cod, Our Lady of the Cape in Brewster, I think, in the year 1983. Or was it 1984? We met on a blind date after I came home from basic training (boot camp). My older sister set us up. It was love at first sight, I think, so if that was in the fall of '82, we probably got married in '83.*

9:01 A.M.

I observe peregrine landing back on church steeple . . .

. . . *I remember the church bell rang for us . . . as I slipped the ring, her band, on her finger. I think the bell rang for the hour, not for us, but a nice touch that I somehow remember all these years later. She still thinks it rang for us and that I planned it that way . . .*

9:41 A.M.

Peregrine still perched. She stretches her leg and her talons open. I'm able to read the band—green over black and numbers 4 over 6. Patience always pays off when observing birds . . .

. . . *When I placed the band of silvery gold on her finger, she spread her other fingers to separate the ringed one from the others. I banded Carol but on the next-to-the-last finger on her left hand. Birds get banded on their legs—sometimes right ones and sometimes left ones. The band was made for her, and it fit her finger perfectly. No extra pushing or second tries. It just slipped effortlessly on her small and well-formed finger . . .*

9:56 A.M.

I know by size and, now, by band number that this bird is a female. This is her hunting perch for the moment. She becomes restless, keeps shifting her position, stalking potential prey with a stealth that defies movement. I see her cock her head, slightly repositioning her body, and then a rush of air as she soars out and nails a pigeon in her talons. She swoops low, then high, bringing the now-limp victim back to the steeple to devour . . .

. . . I feel incredible empathy for the impaled prey, hapless victim of circumstances. Probably never saw the 90 mph blast of feathers and piercing talons that grabbed it, pierced and crushed its diaphragm, squeezed the life out of it, and carried it, limp and lifeless, a fresh kill, back to the perch to eat. I, too, never saw it coming, the four-by-four thrown out from the back of a cargo transport truck, ramming me pretty good in the left side, just missed my eye . . . falling to my knees, weak and semiconscious . . . a victim of war, of a friendly fire jab in the head, of the system, of the fragility of the body in which I live. A war that consumes the very thing it depends on for its lifeblood, the exquisite joy and pain of realizing that we are all victims and victimized, all predators and prey—players on a vast and immutable stage not of our own making, ripe with intangible uncertainty, probability, and always the infallibility of the "I"—wounded by a flying four-by-four or killed by peregrines coming at you from the rear and impaling you right through the heart with talons so razor sharp that they pierce it so cleanly, so perfectly, that not even Dacron can save it; the only thing stopping it from coming right through the breast to the back is its band; bands are good for many things, including marriages and identifying birds from one year to the next . . .

4

The Soft Part Dies

The soft part dies. The hard form stays.
Beauty empty of the animal—
Hush. Listen. It still makes a sound like breathing.
~Kate Gleason, "Chambered Nautilus"

Hawk Watch at Channel 57Q Radio Tower, Manchester
2 October 2009; Cool, Clear, Windy, High 40s to Low 50s F

3:00 P.M.
I set up scope and relax, wait and watch . . . no need to hurry, just need to wait and watch; open up my cooler and eat my late lunch sandwich . . .
   . . . going off to join the army was a big hurry up and wait before I could enter, before there was a slot for me. Nothing about basic was hurry up and wait, though . . .

3:32 P.M.
A raptor flies and perches high up on Channel 57Q radio tower. I identify the individual as a female peregrine. She leaves perch and flies toward, and then under, the bridge across the Merrimack River. She returns with no prey. I note a silver band on her right leg.

3:38 P.M.
Another peregrine joins her, a male by size, hood, and malar stripe. They're perched approximately eight feet from each other on the tower.

3:45 P.M.

I see the band on the male peregrine, black over green, with numbers 6 over 7. He's perched facing into the wind.

3:46 P.M.

I put the scope on the female peregrine and focus in on her band—silver, 02 over 2. I know this pair. I was assisting the Audubon biologist up in the White Mountains when they were banded at the nest site . . . maybe Frankenstein Cliff but not sure.

3:50 P.M.

I watch male peregrine make two sorties in attempts to secure prey. Both times he returns to perch, unsuccessful and with no captures.

4:00 P.M.

I walk toward the tower and look around underneath where birds are perched. I find pigeon remains, head and feathers; they appear stale, not fresh. Perhaps yesterday's kill? Pigeons are a peregrine's favorite food, probably because they are fat and offer a lot of energy per kill.

4:10 P.M.

In my journal I wordplay with the first letters of my name:

R = Raptors and ravens are for Robert, who loves life.
O = Observations in ornithology are for success in science.
B = *Buteos* are big birds that soar through the air, making for a complex web of life—theirs and mine.
E = Endangered and for all those species demanding protection, including eagles.
R = Resiliency, recovery, resourcefulness, redemption, everywhere the birds are, including in my mind's eye, in my heart, and in my body and soul.
T = Talons that tear, capture, pierce prey, squeezing life into death, food for young and old alike.

Talons also act as anchors, balancing the bird on the smallest branch, sheerest cliff edge, and my arm when I am in the rehab cage.

I am contented. *B* is always for birds, bird watching, and my nickname, Bob. *R* is always for Robert, raptors, and ravens. Observing birds, especially birds of prey, such as raptors, sets me free, releases me from me, and gives me a time out. It reduces my limitations and focuses my thinking down to what is right there in front of me—peregrine wings and talons, eyes with bold stares and swivel heads, banded legs stalking prey—the final kill against sky that touches heaven with a sweet updraft of wind and cuts the air with seismic silence, tenses the physical, and then that quick snap of a body grabbed from the reaches of life, impaled within a razor-sharp grasp, prey released into death to nourish predator life. It allows me, the earthbound warrior, a self-inflicted, purely voluntary, and visually stimulating dose of healing grace, amazing grace, an aerial, avian, medicinal RX—and one that has no side effects. I give one last look up at the two peregrines, the female stoically perched, watching as her mate eats his evening meal. I know that as long as they are in the world . . . then so am I.

I look at my watch; time to pack it in and hump down the mountain.

4:20 P.M.

I fold my scope, put it into the car, and head for home, thinking of the poem "Chambered Nautilus," by Kate Gleason. She's a New Hampshire poet. What she writes is true: "The soft part dies. The hard form stays." That's it, then, for the peregrines: they kill and eat, but only the soft part, while leaving the hard part, the bones, the structure and form of their prey, behind. That's true for me, too, in some ways, some soft parts missing, dead I guess, but the hard form, my bones that hold me together, stay on and give me life, give me hope, keep me climbing mountains looking for peregrines. They keep me breathing, keep me from slipping back into the darkened corners of despair even on the brightest of days, keep me feeling and in touch with those I love most, give form to my sockets that protect the soft parts of my eyes. Where would I be without my eyes? Jesus Christ, God Almighty, where would I be without my eyes . . . and my hands, my legs, a moving hip joint, a wrist that bends, a throat intact that breathes the way it should, a head that still functions even with some soft parts missing, retaining its essential form and structure? Where would I be if the hard form was missing and all I had left were the soft parts? Who would I be? What would I be? I know that the wounded soldiers coming back today have body parts missing—legs, arms, hands, feet. I need not wonder what I'd be, for I see my reflection in these absences, solid bodies with no arms, a missing leg, or part of a leg. Same people, different structure. Some even had a face missing that has been put back, sculptured, on the bony form miraculously left behind. War is hell, war is immoral, war is human, war is what it is, and we are the collective collateral paid for the privilege of fighting the good fight.

5

Carrying Guilt

He wanted to "change it up," migrate like birds will,
leave the known behind, find himself where the sun beat
hot, the world was sand, and the people not his own.
~Suzanne Kingsbury, "Peter's Bird"

Peregrine Survey, Mary Baker Eddy Church
on State House Road, Manchester
10 November 2009; Cold, Clear, Breezy, 40s F

10:50 A.M.
I park car and set up scope, begin observations with quick scan of sky
and building tops.

11:00 A.M.
I rescan sky before setting sights on the church steeple. I immediately
detect an adult peregrine perched on top. Observing and then seeing
what's there is all about knowing your target's shape, form, and behaviors.
You have to get inside their skin, their mind, their emotions, and in this
case, their feathers. Like the docs do to me, under and inside my skin.
I continue to keep an eye on the skies and also on the bird perched on
the steeple. Good to know what's happening 360 degrees, horizontal,
vertical, out in front and intuitively what's behind you . . .
   . . . the moment I took my eye off the unloading of those seasoned, dead-
weight beams, the minute I was distracted from the task at hand, my life
changed right in place—past, present, and future collided, collapsed into a

single second, physically and irrevocably. I remember how hot it was, how bright the day was, how dry the air, land, my tongue and lips were. I felt the sides of my mouth crack as the thing cracked into my head; a low, strangled howling escaped from somewhere deep in the lungs where air exchange occurs; eyes shook and life oozed onto the ground, coming out from behind my head and across my face. I remember trying to catch it, hold it back from spilling. I was so out of it that it wasn't until later I was told there'd been almost no blood; the wet stuff was really the bottle of Gatorade I carried, the fruit punch red pooling in watery deep pink near my left ear and across my left check, rolling down my chin and staining my chest. But I could still see out the corner of my left eye. . . .

11:10 A.M.

The peregrine remains in place atop the church steeple almost like a statue placed there to ward off evil demons or roosting pigeons; vigilant and aware; the predator, never the prey . . .

. . . *I couldn't stop myself from being hit by "friendly fire"; damn first lieutenant not aware enough; it had to be me next to him. . . . I am his victim dropped inside the wire, noncombat casualty, wearing the uniform, wounded with guilt, an inglorious injury, invisible wound . . .*

11:40 A.M.

Suddenly the peregrine leaves the steeple, flies northeast out of sight. I can't locate it with my binoculars. Haunt flight? Or hunting flight? I scan the heavens, the blue sky with no clouds. Nothing. I turn to check my watch, adjust the scope, and the peregrine is back on top of the steeple. In less than ten seconds, it came out of nowhere, back to its perch on the church . . .

. . . *But was it my fault? Is it my fault? I carry guilt and the question of why it happened. Whose fault and what ifs stretch taut in me these many years later, even across the turning of a century into another; knitted into the soft parts where hurt and questions weave together in a remembered pattern; the parts that docs or therapists can't reach with knives, scalpels, sutures, hypnosis, or drugs but where nerves, veins, arteries, emotions, thoughts, and the vaporous ache of memory thread through me knots into tension akin to hidden booby traps, trip wires, suicide bombers, a search-and-destroy mission. A slight movement one way or another in thinking or feeling triggers them, and I lie wounded and dying all over again, visceral and real . . . but the guilt I carry matters most . . . and I want to know why. I've heard from other vets, read their stories, too, that the guilt they, I, carry comes from a place that demands external validation for internal wounds. What I know is that those, like me, who are wounded in noncombat operations and have nothing to show for it on the outside tend to carry guilt like a criminal unjustly accused, penalized, because their injuries happened by accident, not by design, not because of some committed action of their own doing, but in spite of it, because of someone else's behavior or condemnation, or something like that. The so-called invisible wounds are those that are least validated by others, as there is nothing to see that says, "I was wounded in the war, in combat, in defense of my country." This may sound ungrateful or self-serving, as we all have relatively intact bodies, but that can be a burden and a blessing when coming home from the war with nothing to show for it yet everything hurting from it. Perhaps I need to express this all to my doctors and therapist . . . or tell them to read this section of the book when it is published.*

11:48 A.M.

A golden eagle soars by overhead. I identify it as an adult. As a cross-check, I open my guidebook and check my identification against the book's description: "Adult Golden Eagles are dark brown with a golden sheen on the back of the head and neck. For their first several years of life, young birds have neatly defined white patches at the base of the tail and in the wings."

11:50 A.M.

Time to go, move out. I take one last look up at the peregrine, fold my scope up, put it in my car, and drive off . . .

. . . I hear my name being called, "Vallieres," as if through a tunnel far off. I'm hoisted up, folded, held in arms not my own. Someone shouts, "Okay, move 'em out, head injury, keep under observation . . . heart, too."

6

Peregrines, Pigeons, Power Towers, and Providence

Look at the birds of the air, for they neither sow nor
reap nor gather into barns; yet your heavenly Father
feeds them. Are you not of more value than they?
~Matthew 6:26

Power Tower Site, Manchester

13 November 2009; Cold, Clear, No Wind, 30s F

2:55 P.M.
I drive, park car, get out, and set up scope.

3:00 P.M.
I scan the power line tower with binoculars first, then scan the sky, then come back to power line tower. I spot an adult peregrine perched on top of tower. No band is visible so I note "unbranded" on the sheet. A closer observation reveals this bird eating prey. Wow, I never get over the thrill of seeing a powerful bird of prey eating its captured prey, a largish bird with webbed feet. No, not webbed feet, wrong angle and light. Now I see that the feet are pinkish, body steel-gray color. The prey is a pigeon, a favorite food of peregrines . . .

 . . . *I was in the wrong place at the wrong time, too bright, bad toss, wrong angle; soldier down . . . food for medics; soldier down favorite food of medics;*

42

but they don't consume you, just parts of you; the rest is salvaged and regurgitated back to the line of duty . . .

4:00 P.M.
I watch, mesmerized, as the peregrine methodically strips its prey down to the essential meal, plies the wings over and over, straining them through its beak until the feathers are gone and bone is all that remains. Sometimes a wing lets go entirely, falls downward, bone and all. Then the mighty beak works the breast, picking off mouthfuls of fine, down-like feathers. I watch as they are gathered by the wind currents and gently carried away, not always downward but sailing away horizontally and in imaginative swirls, twisting and moving, almost dancing in partnership with this invisible force. The strong bill then rips apart the breast and eats the meat there. Lastly, it bites off the head and swallows it whole. Breast and head offer the most energy from a meal per energy expended capturing, defeathering, and eating the prey. Pigeons have a lot of fat and bulk, so they're the preferred meal of peregrines, or at least of the "city peregrines". . .

. . . *strip down, prep for surgery, careful with the head, heart is failing, hurried precision, shave the chest, scalpels at the ready; strong, steady hands rip into breast tissue, cut away and pull out useless parts, toss away . . . prey to surgeons but live to live again . . .*

. . . But humans know the difference, and pigeons being eaten by peregrines do not, they only live to eat or be eaten and reproduce their kind, not to be saved or rescued from their fate because of duty, conscience, or God.

4:30 P.M.
It's cold and dark, so I pack it in. I start the car and look out of the side window, one last glance at life and death and peregrines and pigeons and power-line poles on a frigid day in New Hampshire.

I know how inadequate words are to describe what I just witnessed, how difficult it is to jot down the eternal predator-prey relationship and not project it in human terms, not elicit sympathy and remorse, and not want to rescue the victim of the chase and resultant carnage. I flinch at my own inadequacy at retelling my story. Some things have to be lived at the moment, seen exactly as they occur, self-authenticated by the individual. But even then, our minds, bodies, emotions, and psyches turn it into a singular story and not a universal one. We each must own our stuff, even the parts that happen to us that we're not directly responsible for. Perhaps that's the summing up of life. The birds need no interpretations, justifications, sympathy, or empathy. No surgeries are required for them, no intermediaries filtering happenings. They simply exist. We exist because we think we do. For us to think otherwise is a contradiction of the order of things, of nature, of heaven.

8:34 P.M.

More chimney swifts fly overhead, chattering and cutting the air with their small, sickle-like wings that remind me of peregrines' but in miniature form. Wonder how many more comparisons people have made while observing chimney swifts in the air? I wonder what their habits are—where they nest, how they mate, how long they live, where they migrate to, when they come north and then leave to go back south, how many eggs the female lays, and in what kind of nest? They are charcoal phantoms—almost bat-like in their search for insects, precision gyrations, and seek-and-capture mission. But birds are reptiles and bats are mammals.

8:36 P.M.

I keep watching the aerial ballet, the little swifts pirouetting and prancing across the prenight sky, every so often flicking and flittering across the face of the half-full moon. Suddenly a comet or shooting star zooms across the eastern sky, dropping down over the top of the post office building; it has a long, yellow-gold tail. A wonder of nature right before my very eyes!

I look back up and know it doesn't matter because what I have here is exactly what I am meant to have, and I don't need to go looking elsewhere for what could be. I am managing pretty well with what is. No point in looking somewhere over the rainbow for "better" when better is right here; you just got to live it and appreciate it as it happens for you. And as long as nightjars and chimney swifts ply the airways in this crepuscular time of day, twilight becoming night, I breathe in and out and look up and am contented with half-moons and shooting stars and the birds of this shadowy time of day. No "beam me up, Scotty" for me!

8:48 P.M.

Finally detect a nightjar calling overhead. Now observe many swooping and diving over and around a nearby white-roofed building but still only a single individual vocalizing. Does the white color attract them? Attract the bugs and insects they prey on? Or is it easier for the nightjars to see their prey outlined against white?

8:53 P.M.

Nightjars are small-to-large nocturnal birds that are found around the world, except for the polar regions. Some North American species are named *nighthawks*. Nighthawks tend to have longer wings and tail, and the tail is often notched or forked—however, there are exceptions.

They are sometimes referred to as goatsuckers, as they were often seen in fields together with goats and sheep, and the myth was born that they were there to suck milk from the teats of goats (the Latin word for goat sucker or goat milker is *Caprimulgus*). However, they instead fed on the insects that were attracted to livestock. In the past, night-flying birds—such as the nightjars—were suspected of witchery. Their cryptic appearance blends perfectly into their habitat and they are very difficult to spot during the daytime, when they are usually hidden away sleeping. They are most easily detected at night when light from car headlights reflects from their ruby-red eyes as they sit on tracks or roads. However, their presence is most often made known by their loud calls at dusk. The common names of many types of nightjars are often derived from their call. They inhabit desert regions, grassland and open wooded areas, and forests. They occur from sea level up to thirteen hundred feet, or forty-two hundred meters...

...*Black Hawk helicopter inhabits desert regions, grasslands, open wooded areas, and forests*...

9:10 P.M.

All quiet on the nightjar front. I VHS taped the sound of the single bird but could not pick out which bird was doing the calling. At one point I think I had two different birds calling, one to the southwest of me and one east by south, but no visual detects.

9:20 P.M.

Nightjar diving over white-roofed building. After many sorties, it ends up coming right over me. I lose it after four dives. Then I hear another bird calling from the north. So, two birds, both vocalizing.

9:23 P.M.

Air becomes still and silent, nightjars quiet and invisible. Is this a territory defense—diving and noisy and now quiet? Do they detect and capture prey by sound alone, sally forth according to the direction of the "music of the night"—audible wing beats of moths, biting insects, and other bugs? Or is sight part of the nightjar search-and-destroy mission—where one must die so that the other can live? Captured, killed, eaten . . . consumed.

9:29 P.M.

Observe nightjar sailing quietly over courthouse—seen, not heard. I'm tracking birds by sound and a bit by sight. Nightjars emit a distinctly buzzy nasal sound, "bzeent, bzeent, bzeent," easy to pick out from all background noises. It didn't take me long to learn this call. Night birds are easier to detect because there are not as many birds out at that time.

9:40 P.M.

Nightjar sighted in vicinity of public library. It vocalizes and I track it by sight and sound. Spot it with binos, watch it swoop over library and old state historical society building, but it stays more generally in the linear corridor of the street.

9:49 P.M.

I watch as it lands atop public library building. It sort of does a straight-in landing and puts its feet out just before touching down.

9:53 P.M.

Nightjar up and flying again; vocalizing over library and streaming above street corridor. I lose sight of it a few times while it swoops upward and swoons downward in search of prey—insects—and then it reappears over the library and disappears again.

9:58 P.M.

It's in my sights again, flying and vocalizing—single syllable, "peent, peent, peent," at two-second intervals—then lands again out of sight.

10:00 P.M.

Observe individual flying over library. Are there one or two birds? Mated pair? Nesting on library roof or window ledge or somewhere nearby?

10:30 P.M.

Night observation has run out on me! Nice night out here. Gave out many New Hampshire Audubon newsletters and information sheets about nightjars. Passersby were curious and asked questions, so glad I could hand out info.

I feel good about my observations and wonder why we care so much about these birds that are so hard to see and so hard to keep track of. What purpose besides being part of God's creation plan could they possibly serve? What purpose do I serve, shattered and broken but coming back to life? Seems to me those who want to save all the pieces of God's work, including nightjars, are the closest to understanding God's purpose in creating us and the world in the first place; much more than others who see no value in the entire breadth and diversity of life, who pretend to hold mastery over life and death as a mere human being. Yet those I meet who most want to save the earth and its creatures are not necessarily in alignment with God or even believe in God. Nature spiritualists tell me that they are the ones closest to the earth . . . but not to heaven. Life is a mixed-up place, mixed up like my head, resutured like my heart, crisscrossed like my upper body, full of zigs and zags and rough-hewn scarring. Do we scar inside our bodies like we do on the outside? I have no answer for that question but know that somehow birds sort it out for me; I see them as God perched right there in front of me—creation ordered by night and day, blue and black, gray and white, peregrine and pigeon, small and large, prey and predator; Me.

8

Eagles at the Brewery

Observing birds . . . captivates my mind, challenges
my intellect, and elevates my spirit. They will
continue to do so, because the story is never
over, and there is always more to learn.
~Mercedes S. Foster, PhD, "Manakins and Me"

Winter Bald Eagle Survey, Anheuser Busch
Budweiser Plant, Merrimack
8 February 2008; Silver-Bullet Overcast, Biting Cold, 26°F

11:00 A.M.
Had a good laugh wondering what Budweiser would think of me at their brewery describing the sky overhead in terms of their competitor, Coors! Pull into parking area and set up window-mounted scope; scan with binos.

11:10 A.M.
Looking toward north end of field past the large white pine tree, I observe an immature bald eagle perched in a big white oak tree.

11:30 A.M.
I check the site with prey items placed there by New Hampshire Audubon biologists to ensure eagles have a good food supply to get them through the winter. The prey items, turkey and deer remains, lay buried under

six inches of snow, so I dig up the carcasses and expose them. I note that they arc untouched.

11:35 A.M.
Drive south to the end of the field where the large pines are. Second pile of carcasses is being well eaten but under six inches of snow, so I expose these items as well.

11:40 A.M.
Then walk to other prey items close to river. Note that the immature bald eagle is still perched in the white pine tree south of me. I uncover these prey items as well and expose them; they are well frozen and also uneaten. I observe twenty-five to fifty white birds and fifteen to twenty cedar waxwings.

11:45 A.M.
Worker arrives and begins to work in the yard behind the plant.

12:00 NOON
Two bald eagles soar low and one disappears over the south end of the field toward the plant. Took my eye off the other one to watch this one so not sure where the other eagle went.

. . . That's it, isn't it? We cannot multitask our eyes and our backs, and then things happen like a missed handoff, snap of a head, and pang in the heart that comes out through the back; then two eagles, and I can only pay attention to one and then the other disappears. Difference is, missing a bird doesn't hurt you and lay you low, make you puke up your guts and pee your pants, gulp for air, and have your chest cut open and your heart removed, along with the left subclavian artery and part of your aorta . . .

12:05 P.M.
Scan and catch a soaring adult bald eagle way up north over the river; keep my binos on it as it keeps moving up and away from me over the far tree line and disappears south past the bend in the river . . .

Bend, bends, bent, bending, bended . . . words that slow things like big rivers moving toward the ocean; bends in rivers cut into earth and rock, act like drag on the water that flows along the outside curve but quicken water that flows along the inside curve. I think back to the concept of a boomerang my science teacher in junior high talked to us about, like how the outer curve of the boomerang acts almost as a very slight drag, or rudder, while the inner curve slices through air and quickens the movement, both working in harmony to guide the directional flow of the device through unseen matter—air. I watch the partially frozen river slip between icy edges, water bending to shape the ice's jagged edges; I can almost hear the gurgle and swish, crinkling of ice and water converging, two forms of the same substance meeting, flowing, each retaining its own integrity, two forms undiminished. The curve of my spine compressing against the cage of my ribs, head pressed inward on itself, the curve of my left ventricle slipping on me. Breath shortens, slows, almost stops, almost comes to standstill, then revs up again with new gears in place . . . like an iced-up bend in the river in New Hampshire in the winter. Spring thaw comes and two forms merge into one until the cycle starts over again next winter . . . a heart remade, flesh and Dacron graft, two substances become one, bends intact.

12:27 P.M.

Two more adult bald eagles observed over tree line just north of white pines. I lose sight of them as they fly out over the river. Are these two new birds or the same birds I observed previously, come back together? Are they in the midst of courtship? Time is right for that to happen.

12:33 P.M.

Immature bald eagle takes flight from the white pine at the field's north end, flies over to where exposed prey items are but then turns off inland where power lines are, then drops suddenly down to the ground before reaching the power poles. Why? Is there fresh kill or did it spy a field mouse or other live prey that it prefers over the dead prey put there by Audubon? Did this eagle not see the prey I just exposed? Can't be sure, so I leave notes as mostly questions.

12:46 P.M.

Two red-tailed hawks perched on a branch side by side—a mated pair?

12:55 P.M.

Both red-tailed hawks soar together to middle of the group of tall white pines, near to a small but open water drainage that leads to the river, before I lose sight of them.

1:00 P.M.

Winds are chilling. I turn on vehicle, put window up for warmth, use window mount for scope.

1:05 P.M.

Red-tail perched in white pine, underneath which one of the caches of prey that I dug up lays exposed at north end of field. Red-tail then flies to a small group of leafless trees . . . poplars, I think. So far I have counted seven bald eagles, immature and adult, and two adult red-tailed hawks.

1:10 P.M.

Sub-adult bald eagle observed above power lines soars down to field edge and then disappears behind trees, and I lose sight of it.

1:30 P.M.

I feel the need to get out of the car, stretch my legs. I start walking south about one hundred yards to the bend in the river, then turn around and walk back another hundred yards north. I count twelve Canada geese and ten mallard ducks, two of them males with bright glossy-green heads and yellow bills.

2:07 P.M.

Back in my truck, I move it so I can get a good observation view where I can see some of the river and also north and south views to the exposed prey stations. Snowdrifts are big; four-wheel drive needed. Lots of tracks: turkey, squirrel, chipmunk, deer, otter, fisher cat.

2:10 P.M.

Lunch!

2:17 P.M.

I spy a large flock of the white birds again with black wing bars. What are they?

2:36 P.M.

Two ravens fly to trees above the exposed prey. I look up and see first turkey vulture of the season! The problem with this observation location is that I can't see prey items if a bird flies into the area; can't see if it flies to check out the prey. I decide to move and drive my vehicle north.

3:00 P.M.

I continue driving up the north end of the field and check around the plant's sand and salt shed.

3:44 P.M.

I observe a large flock, again, of those whitish birds with black wing bars putting down on grass. Some land in the tops of trees along the east side of the river. Still have no clue as to what species they are. Wind's picking up; sky is flat gray and seizing up like a frozen radiator. It just feels like all the warmth has deserted the day, been absorbed into a flat plane of nothingness. I lose perspective with no contrast to gauge where horizon ends and snowy landscape begins and now this cold, biting north wind . . . reminds me of lying in the desert sun—made me so hot I sweat cold and shivered; we were warned about heat stroke, sunstroke, heat exhaustion, cold sweats, and no sweat at all—except it's the opposite.

4:12 P.M.

I head down to the river for some protection from the wind. The slight, four-to five-foot drop to the water does the trick and the wind stops attacking me. I count three common and one hooded merganser and take photos.

4:39 P.M.

I walk back up the bank from checking prey cached at river's edge. Winds are howling now. Every piece of me not covered is freeze-dried. I step on ice-covered snow, lifting one foot at a time, and a sharp snap and soft pop follow. It was like summertime down below on the riverbank compared to back up here on the flat of the field: no protective cover and my exposed face hurts. I fight the elements just to get back to my truck.

5:00 P.M.

Do eagles feed during this time of extreme weather? They're not feeding here today as far as I can tell. I see more of the whitish-gray birds, hundreds of them. Wonder what they are? I finally have my bird guide and search the pages for this pretty winter bird . . . and there it is on page 424 in *Birds of North America*, third edition. They're snow buntings!

5:30 P.M.

Day is done, the light gone. Ah, perhaps a faint, lingering pastel glow to the far western horizon. I head home in this cold New England winter weather. I realize I've touched on all three of my favorite disciplines in nature: bird study (ornithology), land study (geography), and tree study (dendrology). The amazing gift of birds is that it takes me to a beer-brewing plant on a cold winter day to see bald eagles flying into trees and landing to inspect prey items cached there by conservationists to help the eagles through a tough winter.

9

Home Station and Back Again

No bird of prey knows that hidden path;
no falcon's eye has seen it.
~Job 28:7

Home Station, Hoit Road, Concord
3 June 2007; Bright, Clear, 65°F

8:12 A.M.
Yellow-shafted flicker, female, noted with head poking out of nest
cavity . . .

. . . *I'm in the army now. I hug my mom, shake my dad's hand (they're
divorced, so this happens separately), and board the plane that will take me
from New Hampshire to Missouri—Fort Leonard Wood, to be exact. Six
weeks and I will be a soldier in the U.S. Army* . . .

8:30 A.M.
A flicker flies from northwest field side and lands near nest tree, perches
for a few minutes, then flies off. Male . . .

. . . *Nothing could've prepared me for the excitement I feel at getting out
of New Hampshire and starting my career in the army. As the plane takes
off, I lose sight of those who are left behind, waving. I suppose my mother felt
like crying but wouldn't do that where anyone could see her. I lose sight of
the ground as the plane pulls up and away, heading south and west. I don't
have time to miss anyone. I'm just into my own present and future, letting
the past slide away for now* . . .

8:47 A.M.

Male flicker flies to nest tree from northeast, pauses, and then flies up to perch five feet below nest cavity. He slowly climbs up to it, looks side to side, and then enters the nest hole. No exit by female observed . . .

. . . *land in Missouri, meet up with my contact who will take me to the military installation. A couple other recruits are there waiting as well. We all look eager but scared. Here I thought I was so full of excitement and now realize I'm really alone and afraid of what's going to happen next.*

9:10 A.M.

Male sticks his head out, opens and closes his beak, then goes back in. I'm uncertain whether young are present . . .

. . . *Fort Leonard fades just as the New Hampshire landscape did six weeks ago, slips into invisibility under the big silver belly of the plane taking me back home for leave. The excitement of being in that state feels stripped out of me. Now I can't wait to be home, eat and sleep in a familiar house, see my girl, Carol, and hope she still loves me like she said she did, hug my mom and really mean it. I start to doze off; head falls forward on my chest, mouth closed, and I hope it doesn't pop open; guys and me joked about that in the barracks; go around shaking salt, pepper, or worse into guys' mouths that popped open when sleeping; watch them wake up, swallow, then run for the sink, spitting and swearing, us laughing . . . hand of the flight attendant shaking me now and telling me to move my seat into the upright position for landing and to make sure my seatbelt is secure around my waist . . .*

10

Aftermath

What wild creature is more accessible to our eyes and ears, as close to us and everyone in the world, as universal as a bird?
~Sir David Attenborough, interview
with Gareth Huw Davies

Peregrine Falcon Observation, Russell Crag Foothills
7 June 2007; Clear with High Clouds, 70s F

8:49 A.M.
Depart home station.

9:46 A.M.
Park car at base of Russell Crag foothills.

10:01 A.M.
Hike to Russell Crag.

11:50 A.M.
I watch for peregrines, but none are visible today . . .
. . . like my wounds. So instead I take notes on myself, do a "me check-in." I try to think back to what I was like before I got injured, but it's hard. I wonder if that part of me, the guy I was before, is gone forever. I remember bits and pieces, they come smattering back into me in small, scattered dots; reminds me of poppy seeds on a bagel or chocolate chips pressed into cookie dough, tiny memory cells sprinkled dark across colorless matter: saying good-bye to Carol, my mom, friends,

calling my dad, how hot it was when we landed in Saudi, why I joined the army in the first place, my heart already wounded by genetics. Then the rapid-fire questions, staccato echoes of bullets hitting targets—would I be sitting here now in nature's solitude, contemplating God's planned next move for me, if I hadn't had an incursion into my head, if I hadn't had a weakened heart but been deployed anyway, doctors who sent me over there because there was not enough time to run my paperwork through the proper channels to get me medically discharged? Hell, I did not even suffer a bona fide war wound, injury came from the incompetence of an officer who took his eye off the ball, so to speak, and threw it at me, hitting me in the head. I'm sure he got promoted anyway and I got disability. I sometimes wonder if it would've been better to have been shot through the head or shot in the heart and died. Is that better than being a survivor and having nothing to show for it, nothing to elicit immediate sympathy from others, but always having to explain the why of my disability, the invisibility of my wounds, the internal carnage safely wrapped inside a skin covering, slicing of the surgeon's knife leaving tracked scars easily hidden beneath a cloth shirt, a heart spliced with the miracle of Dacron?

No one seems to understand a wound they can't see, one that is inside and not outside, one not the result of a bullet or a bomb blast but of a stupid act committed by a young officer. It changed my life, sent me home (not only with a damaged head but with a damaged heart as well) to heal and to learn to live a life with soft parts missing, cartilage twisted like rope, vertebra wrenched out of alignment, and nerve endings and heart tissue simply missing. I have seizures now and depression. I used to have thoughts of suicide, horrific anger, and constant headaches like bombs going off inside my skull. Therapists and doctors tried to help but didn't really understand how it felt to constantly fight a war waged between you and your own body. They haven't experienced the kind of pain that attacks your will and destroys your sanity, your peace, your life force, your will to live. God is the only one who can help when you've fallen into places as despairing as this, for God knows that you're given in life only what you're able to bear. I am Catholic, French Catholic, and learned the Bible from a very young age. Where I grew up in northern New Hampshire, French was my first language. I went to a French-speaking school until I reached high school. Then it was very hard because I had to learn English as my primary language. So I learned then that life is always full of challenges—French, English, God, country, one man down, so many others to fill the slot. War kills, eliminates the very thing that feeds it, gives it life—me, us, you, them. Sometimes I feel as though those armored vehicles in Saudi are driving through my head, rumbling across my nerves, and trying to get my heart to surrender to the peace of dying. But God appears and tells me to press on. Life is not about being safe, protected, uninjured, secure, and free from conflict, pain, and suffering. God tells us that life is a process as full of living as it is full of dying. Life is seeking the grace of God and the forgiveness of self and others. Choices we make affect us if we live to die or die to live. God puts us in situations to allow us to make those decisions and choices, or not, and then we can just give up and let God help us, or just give up.

Head hurts, body drained, brain limp, and I still need to drive home. Must continue to download stuff that's lurking inside the epithelial tissue, though; write it down, document it, keep on keeping on, finishing, fleshing out the aftermath, sort of like a play that ends but the guy comes out after the end of the last act, stands in front of the closed curtain, and talks you through what the ending really means. Except my aftermath has no ending but continues, rumbles on and on and on, no words to say it is over and that it was supposed to turn out a certain way and have a certain meaning; no takeaway message that finalizes it all, wraps it up neatly in a few well-chosen words.

I'm just a mixed-up disabled vet, a jumble of words, trying to figure it all out—after seventeen years and still counting—the skin tag still hanging on me . . . discharged, disabled, rendered inoperable to perform duties as assigned; packed out of the military and sent home; and now what? What is really wrong with me? Or am I okay and the diagnoses wrong? Who gets the last say in whether or not I am disabled? Me or the docs or society? What does that word, *disabled*, mean anyway? How does its definition contain within it the man I am, the man I was, the man I am becoming? Definitions are only words but words that put us in places that give us stuff like a discharge paper or take stuff away from us like opportunities and livelihoods . . . leaving us within the aftermath of the definitions, without direction or sometimes hope.

2:15 P.M.
Still no peregrines sighted. Pack up gear and head back down the trail.

2:52 P.M.
Depart Tripoli Road.

3:38 P.M.
Arrive back home; total of 113 miles round-trip. Good to be home after seeking out the peregrines in their own lair. I know they are well and that they are present in my life but without having seen them today. Faith allows this, makes me heal a little bit more every time I come here, to high places, the haunt of these birds, masters of air and wind, the invisible aspects of life, the essentials of existence.

11

Like Snow in Summer

Masters of the breeze; a Peregrine, a blue-black bullet . . .
swoops low over my truck and disappears; I sit motionless in
the road . . . before I spot it skimming the ridge to my left . . .
cherishing its executioner's mask and spear-tipped wings.
~Jan DeBlieu, "Masters of the Breeze"

Mt. Willard
9 July 2003; Calm, Cloudy, Warm, No Wind, 71°F

1:45 P.M.
I am surrounded by a flurry of down feathers blowing in the wind, around
and up onto the nest ledge and gently tumbling down to where I stand.
Won't see the birds until the heads come up or a feeding occurs or the
soon-to-be-fledged young come out of the crack between the rocks and
start flapping their wings. Amazing how you can be right up almost to
the nesting area and not see the nest or the birds. I set up my scope on
the nest ledge but far enough away that I can make myself invisible to
the birds; immediately observe adult peregrine perched in a dead snag
about sixty feet above the nest ledge.

2:00 P.M.
Train out of Crawford House blows horn to alert it will soon be at bridge
crossing; takes ten minutes until it actually crosses the bridge below
Mt. Willard. Wonder if the train's horn scares birds such as the young
peregrines off nests? Need to find this out. Blue skies opening up above

the mountain; think I need to climb higher to see if I can position my scope at just the right angle to peer into the crevice where the nest is hidden.

2:25 P.M.

I decide to go higher, and as I climb, more down feathers come drifting by me off the nest ledge, white and very small, airy like what I would imagine a baby angel would wear.

3:07 P.M.

I get in a position where I can just see the nest, observe an immature chick madly flapping its wings and creating a snowstorm of down swirling in all directions. The scene makes me laugh. I almost lose my balance, so grab firmly onto a ragged tree trunk, hoping it is sturdy enough to steady me.

3:30 P.M.

I see the same or another of the young poke above the edge of the nest, crown and chest visible; lots of wing flapping and more down swirling in the updraft.

3:32 P.M.

Both immature peregrines are visible!

3:35 P.M.

One of the young is out on the rock on the nest ledge in front of the crevice where the nest lay all but hidden from sight. It does a head bob over and over again; makes me laugh and reminds me of my son Andrew bouncing as he sat on the floor just before he learned to walk.

3:39 P.M.

Both immature peregrines still have down feathers present; both appear alive and well!

3:40 P.M.

They both begin preening and more down feathers come flying out and over the edge of the ledge—like a flurry of snow in summer.

3:41 P.M.

I note a slight size difference in the young—one seems just a bit larger and was probably born a day or two earlier than the smaller, younger one. As I watch the two I note that the older, larger chick has little down left among its feathers, the way my Andrew shed his downiness when a baby and grew the more substantial hair of an adult.

3:44 P.M.

Partly cloudy with breaks of blue sky.

3:45 P.M.

The larger peregrine chick perches on a small outcrop of granite just below the nest ledge but not so far below that the bird cannot easily hop back up.

3:51 P.M.

My peace is disturbed by loud voices down the hill from where I am observing. . . . I hear people talking about my truck, and I immediately run down the path toward it, glad I did not hike too far away. I hear them more clearly saying that the truck is loaded with stuff. They see me and immediately hop on their motorcycles and peel out of the parking lot. I check the locks and all doors are secure. I am a little shaken by this but decide to return to my observation of the peregrines.

4:01 P.M.

I hump back up the trail to the observation point, and the larger chick is still perched out on the rock just below the nest ledge. It continues to preen and fluff its feathers, releasing more down.

4:03 P.M.

I note that this chick has a band on its left leg, silver I think, but in the low light of its perch, I cannot tell. I cannot read it either, so I am missing vital information.

4:04 P.M.

Chick hops back up on nest ledge and disappears from sight. I call it a day and head back to my truck, note that I observed two chicks at about thirty to thirty-four days old, one younger and smaller than the other.

I now process the near-ransacking of my truck by motorcyclists and let my anger come and go; so hard to hang on to it anymore and really hard to do that up here where the peregrines are fledging young and I am at peace with the solitude of this mountainside. Good thing I decided not to hike very far up the slope. Sometimes you only need to climb a short way to make a big difference—both observing young out of the nest and being able to run back down and protect my possessions from theft. Birds steal others' stuff to survive. Why do we steal each other's stuff? I am certain it is not to support our own survival, or is it? God says you shall not steal but we do it anyway . . .

12

Holy Thursday up on the Crag

One seeks God in the things one loves the most. . . .
So, bird watching, that peaceful and seemingly
useless activity, can, in the last analysis, lead us
to God—as every human endeavor should.
~Raul Arias, "Reflections on Bird Watching"

Russell Crag
13 April 2006

A raven pair has nesting success. I see them and hear them "crawing, croaking" that loud throaty gurgle that makes them ravens and nothing more, nothing less, their ungainly stick nest wobbling on the open ledge. But discovering peregrines is my passion up here. I spy the pair, see them fly—dual energy, parallel flights, sharing the airspace as they soar in and out of my sight. I spy a warbler with yellow streaks in the middle of the crown. (I later identify this bird as a golden-crowned kinglet, easily mistaken for a warbler.) A white-breasted nuthatch perches within a few feet of me. I see all this without the use of my binoculars, which gives me a sense of accomplishment in identifying so many species! Shortly, I spot a male peregrine; he flies with ease and stealth among the cracks and crannies of the ledges. He announces his arrival to his mate with a barely audible, high-pitched "aw, aw, aw," a sort of two-syllabic scream, as he unwinds his flight and finds his way into the crag, where he becomes invisible, quiet resides, and the dark must of untold years of nesting here holds the brood. The web of life these birds exist in, depend on for survival, and reproduce within is so complex to me that all I can hope for is that this pair is successful in mating, incubating and hatching young, and fledging the next generation's progeny. I don't see any bands on either the male or female, so I can safely say that they are untouched by human hands here on this piece of earth, holy place, holy day, up here on Russell Crag. It is truly a privilege to see avian life unfold right in front of me, to be able to record that this pair, male and female, is free of human contact. I don't know why that gives me such pleasure but it does. Perhaps the wild in me is satisfied, knowing that it has connected with the wild in these birds and that I am the first to see them as a new pair on this day and on this mountainside. I also surmise that incubation has started, as the male and female are now safely inside the crevice and have not come back out. I suspect they may even have mated again and another egg will soon be laid. The mystery and the unknown, a new discovery, of this newfound pair are what elevate my spirit and call me to come back here again and again. I feel reverential on this holy day, with birds of prey, I pray! God bless the birds of the sky, the mountaintops that reach high to touch the firmament of heaven above, and all of us in whom God is well pleased!

I look down at my feet and find a feather there, only one, and I pick it up and wonder where it came from and from what species.

13

Newfound Pair

Beyond the power of the peregrine . . . the thing
we seek flies elsewhere, remains as music, a dark
silence, becomes water, branches, open sky.
~Macklin Smith, "A Mystery"

Bear Mountain, Hebron, with stop at Hobart Hill
26 June 2007; Muggy, Hazy, 60 to Low 70s F

9:51 A.M.
Depart Concord under a sky full of vapory gray; could almost wring water out of the thick air.

1:00 P.M.
Hobart Hill cliff observations: two turkey vultures swoop and reel; red-tailed hawk flies by; yellow-shafted flicker with crop bulging with food is perched atop a white birch; I spy a pair of young kestrels begging for food as the adults hover nearby; I hear calls of chestnut-sided warbler and white-throated sparrows below where I am perched; a blue jay flies by, melding in color and movement with the azure sky sprinkled with white cloud; I see a mourning dove perched nearby in a birch tree; but no peregrines found here.

1:20 P.M.
Arrive Bear Mountain, Hebron.

1:30 P.M.

I hike up drainage to large crag, scan for target bird—peregrine. I observe one perched halfway up cliff face from my observation point near the large crag outcrop. The bird is sitting in a small birch sapling overhung by a large rock outcrop. I can't tell if it's male or female.

1:45 P.M.

From far right of where peregrine is perched, another peregrine flies in, then circles twice in front of the crevice concealed by the overhanging outcrop before crying out.

1:50 P.M.

She or he then swoops in and lands out of sight. I hear babies begging. A pair tending a nest with young—a newfound pair!

1:51 P.M.

Bear Mountain notes:

I was warned of mother black bear and two cubs; did not observe them.

I was warned of mosquitoes and West Nile virus. Swatted a few dead before they could bite and suck out a blood meal, infect me with their toxin.

I observe one peregrine perched and heard another call somewhere to my rear as I hiked up, that eerie cry that reminds me always of a high-toned whistle or the sound of wind squeezed through a very small space, the thin, vibrational whine that raises goose bumps on my arm.

I am pricked by stinging nettles as a bird let loose its lovely serenade—a Bicknell's thrush identified by voice and location.

I strip down, make a splash in Newfound Lake, and watch the sky above; I see a male scarlet tanager haunt the upper reaches of a white birch, so beautifully attired in orange-red flame and blackened wings against snow-white bark, hedged in green.

See again the peregrine pair, both launched in flight, up here, where they take the show, appear on every channel with no need to turn the TV dial.

I get dressed and descend down, hump it into untouched space as I beat a slightly new and different path back to home.

I claim a good day and confirm this peregrine falcon pair.

14

Scuds and a Paper Death

*The art of war is of vital importance to the State. It is
a matter of life and death, a road to either safety or to
ruin. The Moral Law causes the people to be in complete
accord with their ruler, so that they will follow him
regardless of their lives, undismayed by any danger.*
~Sun Tzu, *The Art of War*

Somewhere in Time

A day void of birds, a day of drab, depressing time, compressing inward, headaches, slight pain as I inhale and exhale. I toggle my pen in my hand; pen takes off in a direction of its own and chases me down on paper. It's a day, like many others, that remains dateless and lost, unaccounted for, empty of will, except for the pen that insists on pressing paper with its fine-tipped point, noting things, lost things, hardly remembered things, that travel along a road rutted and potholed. A narrative flows; a back roads memory more crooked than straight, my story of when I died unfolds on paper, filtered imperfectly, best I can do.

The day arrived when I was released from Walter Reed, one of the chronically wounded, also tagged as GWS (Gulf War syndrome) afflicted. All obvious signs of war were hidden under clothes and skin, cross-wired stitching, looking like a sprung skein of barbed wire flung across my chest and back, cleverly concealed and adjudicated by terms like GWS, temperature stress, PTSD, along with heart, head, and neck trauma;

disabled. I was sent back to Fort Bragg and discharged, officially declared "temperature disabled," and released from duty under that moniker, which simply means, "We don't know what the hell's wrong with this solider, so let's call it heat stress and get him out of here." I think it was the Dacron in my heart causing my body failure and that's why I was discharged, but so much happened it's hard to sort it out. I think now I am considered a head injury, an invisible wound that is not wholly treatable or observable.

So much was wrong with the soldiers coming home from this war. GWS was the new term coined during this war, not invisible wounds or post-traumatic stress or missing body parts due to roadside bombings. No, our wounds were more hidden and secretive, predeployment needle sticks full of vaccines with unknown consequences, all blamed on biological agents that were supposedly spewed across the battlefields in Kuwait, all sorts of body trauma due to rollovers and crazy things like what happened to me, or just plain fatigue at not having been to war before. "Wounded Warriors" was a term yet to be coined and not applicable to us. You see, 9/11 had not happened yet.

The crazy thing is I'd been lost by the army even when I was being treated at Walter Reed. Through a comedy of errors (the mistakes, missteps, miscarriages of command and control, or command un-control), all my records were burned in a building hit by an enemy Scud, and I was lost to the inferno as if I didn't exist and never had. My wife had to resubmit all my records. Then I was told I had to report back to Bragg and reenlist in order to be properly discharged, sworn out on permanent disability.

This was '91–'92. Funny how you can be in a war for your country, then lost to your unit as a still-alive soldier in a bunch of paper piles that burned up in a foreign place that your country deployed you to in the first place via a bunch of papers. Funny how you're considered nonexistent, even as you're injured and medevaced by any number of uniforms who must have recorded your name, rank, and serial number on numerous files and charts. I guess the early part of the last decade of the twentieth century had not yet experienced the computer revolution. (Oh, right,

Al Gore was still an unknown pol and we didn't know him until he was vice president under Clinton, and then we knew, were enlightened, as he told us all that he "invented the Internet." I laugh, thinking that he invented the Internet like he invented global warming. Pols are a kick-ass group of fabricators and prevaricators, and that is just that. I guess we were all paper-pushing Neanderthals before that—the dawning of the age of the Internet.) The pen does this sometimes, shoots off into unintended places, but it makes me laugh when I see what it writes. And me, a lost statistic until I found out my unit called me dead and that made me a nonexistent.

Being declared dead happened after I was transported back home from Germany and sent to a naval hospital in Tidewater Virginia instead of to Walter Reed. In all of that confusion of was I navy or army, I landed in the navy and was left to figure out how to get myself to Walter Reed. I was flown in to Andrews Air Force Base in Maryland just outside DC, then put in a vehicle and driven to a hospital way down in Portsmouth, Virginia—a naval hospital. I was refused treatment once the in-processing folks figured out I was army, a soldier, and not a naval seaman. Somebody in the hospital lobby overheard this mishap and took pity on me and offered me a ride back north to Walter Reed. The ride took hours but I eventually was admitted into Walter Reed a day later. I walked in through the front door all on my own. Carol was there, hysterical. She'd been told I would be there the day before and drove all day to get there, only to find out I was MIA, not there, lost in transition. I was brought back from Saudi for my heart, not my head, although my head still hurt and made me sick and dizzy. It was sort of like a comedy gone wrong or a joke without the punch line: my wife meeting me at the hospital door, crying, me walking in without assistance, checking myself in, explaining who I was, and the whole mix-up. Not until later did I find out my unit had declared me dead. Who really wins wars anyway? If it was all done on paper, no one would, I suspect.

I was dead on paper and alive in the flesh. My life had to be reconstructed. I had to convince the army that I was me and still alive. How does one die on paper and yet live and breathe in the skin one is in? It's almost biblical if you think about it . . . the opposite of the Holy Spirit, really, who breathed life and yet had no corporeal form.

Then remorse, reflection, and a touch of anger set in. I asked myself the ultimate question, the constant replay of the same wondering: Should the army have deployed me in the first place, put me into harm's way with an already-diagnosed aneurysm? That is a question that is unanswerable after the fact. Time and circumstances dictate who goes where, when, and why. I was a solider just reenlisted and was told to report to the battlefield in the Middle East. And I went. It's really as simple as that, except now my body and my heart and my head are full of hurt, confusion, and nerve and muscle pain, a juggernaut of memory that makes me twitch, skewers me in the middle of my eyes, riddles me with confusion and lost hope, makes my wife cry and my son seem unattainably distant sitting right there next to me, while my pen glides along, just trying to make it all permanent. But why? Who cares? The story was written way back then, and nothing can change how it came out.

Why did it happen? How could it have happened? To die and yet be alive in the flesh, to come back to life after dying a paper death, after being Scud-lost in a building bombed and burned somewhere over there, in a Middle Eastern desert (Saudi or Kuwaiti, but does it really matter which?) Again, the unanswerable, how could it have happened? How could a bunch of records burn up over there and take me with them while I was in Walter Reed stateside getting rehab and chatting with my wife? I laugh, thinking I went up in flames. All I can say is war is a funny business: some die, some stay alive, some die and come back to life, some are paper dead and flesh resurrected. Perhaps there is no reality to war, nothing to it but stories, told and retold, written down, vague words tinged by perspective and distance, even wistfulness, the only thing making it all real is having been there, that knowing embedded inside each of us who participated, but truth just maybe seeps in through the retelling of the thing, the experience of just one soldier, or one soldier at a time, who was there, retelling his story, one by one. And the truth seeps out—distilled, sanctified, remembered perfectly imperfect, told to make hearts weep and eyes rendered blink-less, mouths puckered into lips that wrinkle and twist uncomfortably. Isn't that really the point of war, that we who were there can tell stories that make the rest of you uncomfortable?

15

Ode to My Son, 28 August 2007

I dreamed a thousand paths; I woke and walked my own.
~Chinese Proverb

As He Enters High School

My son's first day of high school.
He's becoming a young adult.
I'm honored to be his dad.
Learning to let go makes me sad.
He's maturing in life; I am glad.
His first shave as a young teen
at fourteen; today holds morning dew on the grass.
A promise of life renewing itself as
he walks off to school—son of my morning star!
His life embodies the potential to carry him far.
He is life of my life, gift of birth from my wife!
He is my little peregrine taking flight,
my little fishing buddy and my eye's absolute delight.
Andrew, you are fledged and I must try
and let you go, watch as you flap and fly,
glide all on your own, resurrection of life divine.
I only hope I've made all the difference in your life as you have
    made in mine.

16

Ode to My Son, 3 October 2007

Poetry is like a bird, it ignores all frontiers.
~Yevgeny Yevtushenko

On the Day You Were Born

A decade and a half ago you were born
and I rejoiced, your mother rejoiced!
Now today is the day of your fifteenth turning.
You were born in the season called fall,
your colors illuminating us all.
You're our gift, your presence among us.
You bring happiness to us all.
Born in this season called fall.
The day you were born, I walked on air.
The gift of who you are I want to share.
Although skies may turn gray, your smile
is that ray of light shining through.
You are more than I can say!
You're the sunshine, you're the springtime,
you're the snow that falls; you're born unto us—
the greatest and best gift of all—
heaven's heart in me!

17

Ode to My Son, Reflections

*My little sisters, the birds, much bounden are ye unto
God, your Creator, and always in every place ought ye to
praise Him, for that He hath given you liberty to fly about
everywhere, and hath also given you double and triple
raiment; moreover He preserved your seed in the ark of Noah,
that your race might not perish out of the world; still more
are ye beholden to Him for the element of the air which He
hath appointed for you; beyond all this, ye sow not, neither
do you reap; and God feedeth you, and giveth you the streams
and fountains for your drink; the mountains and valleys for
your refuge and the high trees whereon to make your nests;
and because ye know not how to spin or sow, God clotheth
you, you and your children; wherefore your Creator loveth
you much, seeing that He hath bestowed on you so many
benefits; and therefore, my little sisters, beware of the sin of
ingratitude, and study always to give praises unto God.*
~Saint Francis of Assisi, *Sermon to the Birds*

To cocreate a new being is to offer hope to the world when you feel all
hope is gone, to look at the miracle of life with wonder and awe, to blink
and still see the amazing grace of your life combined with another's into
a new being, nature at its finest. If only we could always and forever
hold on to this first-time amazement, this offer from God that life super-
sedes our existence and is recombinant in a baby born this day. He is
mine and Carol's, ours only until the day he becomes his own man. We

are caretakers of this divine inspiration until we know to let go, always hopeful that he will want to come back sometimes and visit, come back to his place of birth, his childhood roost, and stay a while. Just with his presence, he takes me to the heights of a peregrine aerie, the deep and craggy, invisible place where babies are born covered in down and with bones more like hollowed tubes than marrowed core. Stay in my heart always, son of mine. You are the stuff dreams and hopes and futures are made of. I give you to the wind and mountains and remote cliff edges. I launch you off into life like a peregrine launches her young off the rugged cliff edge. Fly high, strong, and with purpose of goodness. Stay as safe as you can for as long as you can. And go as far as you can go, always with God's grace in your heart. You are always in mine.

18

The Call of God

Then I heard the voice of the Lord, saying,
"Whom shall I send, and who will go for Us?"
Then I said, "Here am I. Send me!"
~Isaiah 6:8

Peregrine Watch, Downtown Manchester
3 March 2008; Cloudy, Cold, Raw NW Wind, 41°F

12:15 P.M.

I sit in my car with the heat on and scan along edges of buildings lining Elm Street. I scan the street and almost immediately I spy a pair of adult peregrines perched on the opposite edges of the Public Service of New Hampshire building—the smaller male is perched on the southwest corner of the top of the building and the larger female is perched on the northeast corner.

12:17 P.M.

Male takes to the wing, flies east, banks south, lands, and perches on the southwest top of building. Female does same but flies southwest, banks, circles, and does a large sweep low across the sky, lands, and reperches almost in the exact spot that she took off from, northeast and diagonally across from where the male is perched.

12:20 P.M.

I drive over to Concord Street for better view of peregrines and the public service building. I scope male and see band on his left leg—black over green, 6 over 7.

12:25 P.M.

Male does another takeoff and landing, perches back at the southwest corner.

12:59 P.M.

Female does another flyover and this time swoops close to male.

1:07 P.M.

Female calls, turns and faces north; she is also banded.

1:11 P.M.

Two crows fly through peregrine falcon observation area. I wonder if we ever band crows.

1:15 P.M.

Female leaves perch and flies north to bridge; soars and swoops from side to side, then returns to perch on the middle northeast rail of the power tower.

1:20 P.M.

She shifts her position and faces directly north.

1:27 P.M.

She turns her entire body several times in a few minutes' time. I wonder if she's hungry, looking for prey, or just vigilant. Belly band appears a peachy color.

1:30 P.M.

My observations are over for today and I get into my car and drive home, knowing I've answered the call of the wild, the call of God to go forth and understand myself through the observation of these majestic, pliable, flexible, and emotionally stirring birds of air and land. I want nothing more than to simply serve these birds and to serve God, to find myself, my meaning, my purpose under the same sun that these birds claim as their own. I want to find in the nature of things, the watching and the writing down of the smallest details, always attention to detail, the very essence of the thing that will unwrap my pain and assuage my anger, making it melt away.

The more I learn about these birds, the more I learn about myself—and the more that is revealed to me in some unseen way. The birds relieve my stress, ground me, and make me feel alive, give me a reason to get up in the morning and come back home again later in the day. They subdue my headaches and quell the depths of my well-protected, perhaps even well-fed, rage. They teach me truth and justice and the ultimate necessity for simple survival, that doing battle every day is part of that, and so is struggle for what sustains us, even to kill or be killed in the process.

I wonder as I sit here in my truck, binoculars snugged in next to me around my chest and partly over my heart, what if we handed out binoculars instead of guns and the war was won by the side that counted the most birds in a single day? It could be a "Big Day of Birding" instead of a "Big Day of Slaughter." But then I wonder, are two peregrines the equivalent of a thousand pigeons? Or twelve human lives? Or a gaggle of geese that some see more as food than as an eyeful of delight? Always, then, the eternal question of the value of things, those sacrificed and those doing the sacrificing, those that eat or those that are eaten, those that shoot or those to be shot, deciding ultimately who wins or loses.

What nature teaches me most is that there's not a determination of winning or losing. It is simply about survival; nothing else matters. Or does it? I think the way we as humans decide to survive does matter, and matters most of all to us and our humanity. Do we always want to kill each other, be at war, be hurt by another human being, live and die ungrateful and unaware of God's divine love and grace? Perhaps this is all best sorted out in one of my favorite Bible passages, put to music back in the day by the rock group The Byrds and included here for clarification of just how hard things are to sort out for one guy with a love of birds, a shredded heart, a confused head, and a deep and abiding faith for the way things are:

> For every thing there is a season, and a time for every purpose under heaven:
> a time to be born, and a time to die;
> a time to plant, and a time to pluck up that which is planted;
> a time to kill, and a time to heal; a time to break down, and a time to build up;
> a time to weep, and a time to laugh; a time to mourn, and a time to dance;
> a time to cast away stones, and a time to gather stones together;
> a time to embrace, and a time to refrain from embracing;
> a time to seek, and a time to lose; a time to keep, and a time to cast away;
> a time to rend, and a time to sew; a time to keep silence, and a time to speak;
> a time to love, and a time to hate; a time for war, and a time for peace.
>
> *~Ecclesiastes 3:1-8*

19

Eagles on the Island

No man is an island entire of itself;
every man is a piece of the continent, a part of the main . . .
any man's death diminishes me,
because I am involved in mankind.
And therefore never send to know for whom
the bell tolls; it tolls for thee.
~John Donne, "Meditation XVII"

Bow Lake Eagle Survey, Strafford and Northwood
24 October 2007; Warm, Sunny, Clear, 60°F

11:12 A.M.
I turn onto Fire Road 38; I find the kayak, blue with white paddles, laying on the gravelly shoreline in front of the cottage. I have the right place, the one owned by the Audubon volunteer who said I could use his kayak.

11:15 A.M.
I slide the boat halfway into the water, load it up with my gear, and then step into the scooped-out plastic body. I slip into the seat and push with the paddle until I am gliding free of the shore, cutting my own path through silently still water; me, a small fish on a big lake in a long narrow boat with a paddle for wings—I am winging my way on the surface of the water . . .

. . . Life is like that a lot of the time: you just wing it, hoping it all works out, like joining the army, getting married, having children, picking up the

pieces of life after tragedy—but more, knowing that there are still pieces to
do something with—finding your own way through a fog of partial body col-
lapse and inability to do anything about it on your own, the terrible sense
of separation from self and the ones you love, more like severed isolation
without the absolute physicality of something blocking you from the other.
Now only nature, and mostly birds, break down and melt away that feeling.
The feelings, like islands, floating free around inside of me, with no anchor
and no keel to direct them where I want them to go . . .

11:30 A.M.

I start paddling northeast to the far rocky shoreline. I lay my paddle
lengthwise across the kayak and press my elbows on its handle to steady
myself as I scan the distant shoreline with my binoculars. Nothing pops
into view, so I paddle in and out of undulating coves, convex points of
rock and ledge and concave bays of mud and weeds that define the
shoreline's individual topography. I then skirt around the nearby islands
where past recons indicated bald eagles nesting. I pause and cross myself
with the paddle again for a steadier view and spot a possible stick nest
on the most isolated of all the nearby islands. The island sits twenty to
thirty feet in front of me and hangs just barely off the mainland shore,
but not near any other islands and in the remotest and most undevel-
oped part of the lake's shore. The nest rests in a large white pine, near
the top, and secured within a tangle of branches. If the light wasn't just
right, I might have mistook the garbled mass of greenish-brown for
witches'-broom, a misfiring in the normal growth of a plant caused by
any number of things, including funguses, diseases, insects, viruses, or
improper pruning. Not unlike my brain now, a garbled misfiring due to
any number of reasons, but mine is due to abnormal behavior by a young
officer that caused improper functioning acutely and now chronically.
It happened a very long, long time ago, but memories seep in when the
present-day visual offers me a clue to remembering.

I uncross myself from the paddle and glide closer to the island, where
I see several ravens lurking near the nesting tree. I quickly move into
position around the left side of the island and take a photo. I take note

of the fact that Bennett Bridge is an obvious shoreline feature directly north, or at twelve o'clock, from the island and pretty much points at the nest tree. With my binos, I scan the other trees on the island and don't observe any eagles. I decide to check out another island about sixty feet from the nest tree island and paddle slowly and quietly over to its shore, a brown, soft mud punctured by a few rock faces held above the waterline. I beach my craft and step out onto squishy, semisolid ground. I quickly discover that it is much easier viewing from the kayak than from land, so I relaunch. As I paddle around the island, I finally observe two adult bald eagles perched together in the top of a white oak. I watch them for a while but they seem content to remain perched and unmoving. Could this be the pair that used the stick nest on the nearby island?

11:50 A.M.

I paddle away from this end of the lake and move south, where there is more development and less wildness. I give the passing shorelines occasional scans and note that the beach on this side of the lake is heavily eroded and is fenced off in places, perhaps due to the many powerboats docked in front of the cottages and houses along this stretch of lakeshore. I scan all the trees, looking for last year's nest, one that a lakeshore resident reported to Audubon as having eagles in it last spring. I detect a nest, land based and not island based, but no bald eagles nearby. Perhaps the pair I saw earlier used this nest. I don't know, and there's no way I can determine that now.

12:18 P.M.

I'm hungry and decide to eat while on the water. I haul in the paddle, drop it inside the boat, and just float. I have become an island, just hanging out on the water, surrounded on all sides by a matrix that will not support my own weight, which could drown me by filling my lungs with water and not air. How ironic that the element that can quench my thirst and keep my body alive could also kill me. Life is full of these opposites, polarities, and conundrums.

12:40 P.M.

I turn and head back toward the big island where I discovered the eagle nest. As I get closer, I look at the top of the white pine and now the pair of bald eagles is perched in a nearby pine tree. I again cross myself with the paddle and decide to pull out my window-mount birding scope. I steady it on the hull of the kayak, pull out the small tabletop tripod legs, and capture both birds in a single view. A smooth jolt of electricity goes through me, not the kind that makes you jump but the kind that reaffirms and gives you a deep satisfaction at completing the mission . . .

. . . *the taut-nerve, almost palatable feeling that sucks at your mouth and draws moisture from your lips when you are reconning and your heart's racing and your breath comes quicker but you will the body still and make your eyes focus in the gray fog of war . . . wondering, wishing, hoping you will see it (or them) before it (or they) sees you . . .*

1:00 P.M.

A fish jumps out of the water thirty yards to my left front, a slight spray following as the fish dives back into the deep. I turn the kayak, head directly to the island, and drive the kayak up onto a small beachhead jutting between granite jags—long, low slabs of rock that seem to slide off the island and into the lake like lava flowing from a volcano.

1:19 P.M.

I'm out of the water and up on dry land. I watch one of the adult eagles preen and poop. Another word for this act of waste removal is defecating, but poop just seems appropriate and more understandable. Now I can see both from the bottom up, good looks at both sets of legs—no bands encircle the legs of either of the pair! I jot this discovery down in my notebook.

1:57 P.M.

I shove off from the island and start slowly wending my way back across the lake.

2:01 P.M.

I hear common loons yodeling and watch as one of them paddles madly with its webbed feet across the surface of the lake and finally lifts off and takes flight out of sight. I sense that these loons still in New England in late October are probably fledged young from this year's nesting. Adults usually migrate south weeks before the young; thus my supposition that these are young birds and will soon be winging their way south as well.

2:09 P.M.

I keep my eyes and ears alert as I slowly paddle my way back to my launching spot. I hear crows and look to my right and see a bald eagle soaring way up high over what I believe is Tasker Hill, a small, short rise on the shore side of the western edge of the lake. I also note a gaggle of thirty or more crows flying underneath it, acting like an escort, a very noisy, squabbly chorus.

2:21 P.M.

I reach the beach in front of the house and gently deposit the kayak back where I found it, overturned and lying on the rough, gravelly beach. I sit on the grass and tally my observations for the day:

> Two adult bald eagles roosting near the nest on "Big Island"
> Heard loons and observed a single loon lift off and fly away
> Observed a handful of turkey vultures soaring over lake
> Counted numerous common crows, including the thirty or so "escorting" the bald eagle away from lake
> Identified a single yellow-rumped warbler
> Noted three ravens
> Heard but did not see many black-capped chickadees

2:35 P.M.

Before leaving, I turned for one last look out across the lake at the islands jotting its surface. Driving home, I begin thinking that islands are whatever isolates something from something else or someone from another—land from water, earth from sky, ocean from shore, continents from other continents, people from each other, dead from the living, a baby from its mother, a diagnosis—which can be a negative or a positive, but where positive means negative things and negative means positive things: a positive diagnosis means you have a problem and a negative diagnosis means you don't. I had a positive diagnosis and was discharged, cut off from the normal way of doing things. Even my driving my truck alone separates me from the outside and is like riding shotgun alone, an island unto myself, windows rolled up tight and me the only driver.

20

They Steal My Blood and Sanity Sometimes

Little fly,
Thy summer's play
My thoughtless hand
Has brushed away.
~William Blake, "The Fly"

Russell Crag
23 May 2012; Clear, Cool to Warm, 60s F

4:00 A.M.

The scream of a 4:00 a.m. alarm always reminds me of being in the military. No matter how many times over how many years, rise and shine at 4:00 a.m. is hardwired into me. I relax and fall back on my pillow. But I know I have an hour's drive ahead, so I sling one leg and then the other off the bed, followed by a more-resistant body. In less than twenty minutes I'm in my car, driving north. I watch the earth wake with the sun shining after literally weeks of rain. It's a catharsis of the soul, an epiphany of the spirit, tonic for a pent-up bird-watcher always with an eye toward spring and the thrill of migration and nesting season for the peregrines. I travel the same route as I have before, taking mental note of the season's progression and of things like leaf out of the trees and the height of the grass along the highway as well as the color of the sky.

5:15 A.M.

I arrive at base camp, park my car, and gather my pack, binos, insect repellant, hat, sunglasses, notebook, water, and lunch.

5:20 A.M.

I begin my ascent, walking up the well-tended and relatively flat trail that takes me to the next level—a set of steep, much narrower, and less well marked trails. Many times before I have had to figure out which way to go and have had to blaze my own trail, slashing through overgrowth that clings, claws, and sticks to my skin and clothing.

6:00 A.M.

I stop along the trail where the flat smoothness narrows into sinewy curves. I lean against a big rock that marks the change in landscape and watch as streamers of sunlight illuminate spaces between leaves and trees. I take a drink of water, swat black flies that swarm me, and haul out the bug spray. I shoot it at them and then coat my arms and clothes. I turn the can over and read the warning: "Contains Deet, don't spray directly on exposed skin" . . .

. . . *we are in a toxic waste dump with stuff that smells, clings to the inside of your nostrils, drifts to the back of your throat and makes you cough, choke, puke, dry heave poison dust laced with a filmy something not quite liquid and not quite powder. But in the end you swallow anyway; there is just no way out of this place, full of things carried here, thrown away, buried and left behind by the enemy. Then we come to defend it because someone decided it was a safe haven from attack . . . and our eyes tear and burn, and our hands itch and our porous uniforms lay on our bodies like toxic sieves, letting it all in but not letting it back out, skin breathing it all in but not perspiring it back out . . . in this desert of waste where it's all dangerous, all out in the open, exposed . . .*

7:09 A.M.

Humping up the steeper, narrow trail, I need to stop and rest. I find a nearby rock, sit, and have a drink of water and pop a peanut butter cracker in my mouth. I've come to hear the call of the wild, waiting for the winds to pick up a little to keep the damn black flies away. They steal my blood and my sanity sometimes . . .

. . . just like the war did, and some of my flesh and bone, as well as half my heart, too . . .

The war memories shake me to the core. I can't control their comings and goings. I shake loose from them and refocus, which is easier to do now that I have birds and New Hampshire hot-wired into my being.

7:14 A.M.

Up and moving again. I pass an old miner's camp. (Is this the one I noted last year?) It has left its mark—an abandoned chink in the granite fabric of this mountain. I remember reading somewhere that New Hampshire had graphite mines, and I wonder if this is what the miner was seeking. Everything up here seems small compared to the mass of this mountain, even this minor tear in the granite chipped away at by an unknown miner long ago. Even me, even the peregrines that I hope to find farther up the climb.

7:50 A.M.

I reach my observation point, sit on the edge of the rocky ground, and look up and out. I watch blue jays as they pick and prod their way up the crags, looking for grubs and other bugs. I wonder if the peregrines would catch jays as prey. A raven family is nearby, the adults feeding the young in a large nest up on an open ledge near where I suspect the peregrine falcons are raising their young deep within a hidden crevice. I'm blessed, sitting here in a National Forest jungle in the White Mountains of New Hampshire, gobbling up its beauty, an ever-changing scene of natural succession. I listen as ravens call, then warblers, thrushes, and nuthatches.

In this place I find peace. It's remote, wild, and extreme. I wait for the peregrine to come out from deep within the crag. I love birding's attention to detail . . .

. . . attention to detail is how my life was saved and my heart rebuilt. They went deep within the crag of my chest and cut away the bad stuff and replaced it with surrogate synthetic stuff. The rest was up to me—live or die . . .

8:00 A.M.

The peregrines are not at last year's nesting ledge. They're not at the ravens' large stick nest near the top of the ledge overhang. Then I see them, two wild peregrine falcons without bands on their legs! Both are adults and they are perched on a ledge outside a horizontal crag near two white birch saplings . . . stark white bark against a gray-black background.

8:05 A.M.

I hump hard over the rocks to get to a closer observation point. I hear the peregrines—in a food exchange and also a feeding, I think. But I'm climbing too hard and fast to stop. I need to get to the observation outpost ASAP.

8:15 A.M.

Pair of peregrines confirmed! They act agitated, and I realize I have on a white shirt. I quickly change into a charcoal-colored one I carry in my backpack. Their agitation stops. I blend better now with the shadows, rocks, and shadings of the surroundings—my birding camo!

. . . camo in the desert is beige, just beige and shades of beige. Always good to blend in but never any cover, shade . . .

8:17 A.M.

I settle into my new observation niche and watch. What a privilege it is for me to be here, to bear witness to such a hidden work of nature. Am I the first to see this pair? To record that they are not banded? I will acknowledge that I spotted them first, found their nesting hideaway, and recorded that they carry no bands . . .

. . . I am married but my fourth finger on my left hand no longer carries my band, the band my wife placed there when we married . . .

But that happened a long time ago, when I was injured and came out of surgery. My band was missing but later returned to me. I look down at it now and twist it around my finger. Bands do carry significance, and we like to denote pair bonds by banding, whether it is birds or ourselves.

8:40 A.M.

I sit in silence, soak in the healing concoction of cool, clean air fragranced sweet with pine and fir and the very alive smell of decay. Why does decay in the north woods smell so alive? Makes me want to gulp it in. I'm not sure there are words to describe what I am feeling, but the closest I can come to it is this: after a really bad rainstorm in the summer in New Hampshire, the sun comes out from behind a dark cloud that attaches to a white cloud and the sky is blue and black and the rain has just barely stopped falling and then a rainbow appears . . . you are so alive in that moment that you live for that rainbow, you give in to it and merge with it and you gulp it, gasp for its air and its reason for being, and life is that perfect and that revealed. Sometimes soldiers tell me adrenaline rushes through them like that when they are on a mission, when they pull the trigger to kill the enemy, when they return to base camp pumped up and ready to roll all over again even though they are dog tired and can hardly stand straight. I hear ravens call way below me . . .

8:46 A.M.

. . . and then watch as a raven, with prey squished in its beak, announces its return to the nest. One of the peregrines watches as I watch and suddenly dashes downward toward the raven and harasses it. I wonder if it harasses the raven because it is too close to the peregrine's nesting territory or if the peregrine wanted what the raven had clutched in its beak. I watch, fascinated—reality unfolding, unedited, unscripted.

8:50 A.M.

One peregrine remains perched on the horizontal crag near the white birch sapling; the other peregrine detaches from its harassment of the raven and perches far below the other peregrine on a rock shelf leading into the crag where I suspect the nest is.

8:57 A.M.

The peregrine perched on the ledge near sapling birches walks back into the deeper hollow of the ledge and disappears out of sight.

9:15 A.M.
Ravens call. Now is the patient part of birding and the intense, focused observation. I get up and stretch before settling in for the stealth mission—close and constant observation of the ledge where the peregrines have their nest.

9:35 A.M.
A peregrine down below flies in and out of the crevice where I suspect the nest is.

9:50 A.M.
The bees are buzzing. I pick a tick off my arm.

10:35 A.M.
Pileated woodpecker calls down below. I also hear winter wren, black-throated blue warbler, red-eyed vireo, and black-and-white warbler. Ears are a good thing to have when birding . . . eyes, too, but ears are a must. No eyes would leave me dependent on another to climb here, so all in all, good to have both.

10:55 A.M.
Pileated calls again—a hauntingly shrill scream, deep and resonant, echoing through deep temperate forest and granite crag.

10:57 A.M.
Ravens carrying food fly into nest to feed young! I love doing this. It's hard, but to be with nature is how I find solace now, peace with myself, my world, my life, and my life before birds when all I wanted to be was a career soldier.

11:01 A.M.
I call it a day and pack out.

21

Three-Quarters of the Way up Eaglet Spire

Most High Glorious God
Enlighten the darkness of our minds
Give us a right faith, a firm hope and a perfect charity
So that we may always and in all things
Act according to your Holy Will
Amen.
~St Francis of Assisi, Vocation Prayer

Eaglet Spire, Three-Quarters of the Way Up
22 April 2010; Clear to Cloudy, Cool to Cold, Windy, Low 50s F

10:30 A.M.
Arrive at base and begin ascent. Stop halfway up and then continue until I observe peregrines. I find a good observation point and stop approximately three-quarters of the way up the spire.

11:50 A.M.
An adult peregrine flies out from within a hidden crag, calls, and then flies toward what is commonly called Eagle Cliff, to the south side of the spire. Another adult peregrine flies after it. They soar together, with one positioned slightly above and to the right of the other one.

12:05 P.M.

The obviously larger female returns to spire ledge and chirps, then walks into the crag and out of sight. The smaller male lands at the same spot as the female, pauses, but does not enter the crag. Instead, he takes off again and disappears around the back side of the spire. I have confirmed a pair and what appears to be a nest hidden within the rock crevice.

12:10 P.M.

All is calm, and I decide to move to a different observation location on the other side of the spire. I want to see if I can locate last year's failed nest ledge location. I see some whitewash on the ledge, but there appears to be no active peregrine nesting activity. On closer inspection, the whitewash is dull and discolored, not fresh, and I am now certain this nesting site is not being used this year. I return to the active nest ledge and my previous position. I decide not to post any Endangered Species Nesting signs at the unused nest location. I make myself comfortable, pull out my lunch, and watch for additional peregrine movement.

1:01 P.M.

Wind picks up and I feel cold and clammy. I hear a peregrine calling from within the spire nest area.

1:17 P.M.

My feet are soggy and I need a change of socks—soaked from sweat and a misty rain that has just begun.

1:32 P.M.

I've added another layer of clothes, wind gusts biting. It feels like snow. I need to find cover where I can still see the nest ledge . . .

 . . . *shelter from the sun, cover from the relentlessness of too hot, too bright, too barren; need a change, a change of anything, including desert camo that makes the scene all too cryptic, like you can hide right out in the open and be missed by a passerby, if there ever were such an event. . . . God, not even a rock or tree for as far as the eye can see. Who would live in such a place as this? What makes them stay?*

1:34 P.M.

I reposition under a large overhang with just the right angle for me to set up my scope, just in time to see the male peregrine fly by in front of me and disappear over one of the small jagged outcrops, a stalagmite-like formation, on the eastern slope of the spire. Immediately after he flies, I hear the female calling and the male calling back.

1:42 P.M.

The male peregrine is up again and flies from behind the east edge of the spire. It is carrying prey secured in its talons, then lands on the middle cliff below the nest ledge, where I lose sight of him. I wonder if the prey is his dinner and not his mate's. It begins to rain, a cold, chilling rain with temperatures dropping, but I don't want to leave yet . . .

   . . . here the sun sets and the temperature drops from 120°F to 100°F. I feel better now that everything is black and nobody sees anything. It erases the brain tease of the day, when you somehow think you can make water and greenery appear just by wishing it, or missing it, so badly that senses fool what the eye denies . . .

2:10 P.M.

The female calls from within the nest ledge. I need to post an Endangered Species Nesting sign along the cliff face around this nest ledge, which means I have to climb up and down the slick rock faces. I look at my watch and realize time is running out for my observations of this pair, and I have three signs to put up. Plus, conditions will be bad on the descent.

2:30 P.M.

Signs hung and I am safely back under cover of the overhang. I'm wet and tired, so I pack out. I've had the amazing privilege once again of confirming a nesting pair of peregrines. I wonder about people who go off to jobs every day and if they feel as privileged and as satisfied as I do at the end of their day? I don't get paid for this work; I volunteer and often wonder if that's what makes all the difference.

4:15 P.M.

Arrive back at my car and give one last look up before I turn and drive away . . . yes, sometimes going only part of the way up is good enough . . .

 . . . *partial recovery, never fully operational again; Dacron causes bacterial infections and other complications. You cannot perform your duties, you will be discharged disabled. Oh, yeah, discarded as if I was never really there. Being able to heal only partway is not good enough for the army to keep me on. I accept that. It's all about being able to carry a gun, go off to war, and fight the enemy on their own ground . . .*

22

Backside Slide

*Heaven makes heard the glory of God and the
firmament shows the work of his hands. . . .
The heavens declare the glory of God, and the
sky displays what his hands have made.*

~Psalm 19:1

Eaglet Spire, Backside Slide
26 April 2010; Mostly Clear, Warm, 60s F

12:41 P.M.

It's Earth Day and I celebrate
this life of mine, so precious and divine,
as I ponder peregrines' future issue; see them
fly deep within the crumbly gloom, the womb
of carved rock, a cave, where they mate and lay
their eggs, young soon to hatch, fledge them, too.
It's clear today as I climb to set my scope on level ground
and view mighty birds of prey reveal their magnificence!
My struggle to reach this place, where time has worn its face
on jagged, deeply lined, and unhumbled space, where it is
so very cold I add another layer; slip icy fingers into gloves.
Just another spring day, a chance to peer into
heaven's gate, and all I need to do is to keep moving,
just moving around, to stay warm and know that I am alive.

2:20 P.M.

I am exhilarated to come back here and check on last week's confirmed pair of peregrines. I hiked up a different route this time, actually one I made myself (sort of my road never traveled), and on the day Earth proclaims as its own. I immediately observe a peregrine fly out from the spine of the spire that hides the nest from my view. I hear peregrines calling from behind me and turn just in time to see both male and female.

2:52 P.M.

I post the cliff edge with more Endangered Species Nesting signs here and jokingly pin one on my chest. I read it upside down and then remove it and nail it on the small white birch sapling about fifty feet underneath the nest ledge. I always wonder why humans cannot be endangered as well as birds. We are things like ADD, ADHD, PTSD, GWS, disabled, visibly wounded, invisibly wounded—sanitized by words distilled into an essence of just a few letters, made small and nothing like being the larger word "endangered." Maybe it would be better to just call us all endangered and we would be cared for and looked after in a different way—a better way, perhaps, but no telling really. Sometimes I feel like a footnote to humanity.

3:09 P.M.

I see the male peregrine perched now on the middle cliff just above me, no band on either leg. Its back is slaty gray and its chest has extensive horizontal barring. With so much beauty before me, it is hard for me to stop the tears. I am so lucky, fortunate, and thankful for the opportunity to work with these birds and really get to know them in the wild places where they spend their lives.

3:15 P.M.

I observe and sketch this bird, then hike down.

4:05 P.M.

Back at my truck, I look at the image on paper and then close the cover of my notebook. I head for home with the peregrine tucked safely by my side.

23

Square Ledge

When we rise in the morning, we give thanks for out of the
sky land there emanates . . . Sky Beings . . . giving to our
lives and our work countless and unending days of joy.
~David F. "White Buffalo" Hayes, "Joys of the Day"

Square Ledge
9 June 2010

1:00 P.M.

I've made it here today into Mountain National Forest. The Old Man of
Square Ledge silhouetted, embedded way up there, hanging in profile
off the shear granite face. It's a cool June day and the black flies are
biting viciously. As I sit to have lunch, I notice the remains of a blue
jay's tail, the rest of the bird eaten by a peregrine, I presume. Just as
I write these notes down, my first sighting of a peregrine occurs—an
adult bird swooping down and into a hidden crevice where I lose sight
of it. I listen intently and hear the squabbly begging of young birds in
the nest. I heave a big sigh of contentment, open my lunch bag, and
look around me.

I see bluebirds at the nest box at the edge of the field at Franconia
Road. Also yellow-shafted flicker and tree swallows. My dad's favorite
butterfly flutters by and lands on an as-yet-unopened thistle plant—a
big, beautiful, yellow-and-black-striped tiger swallowtail.

After lunch I sit, wait, and listen, trying to determine more precisely where the peregrines have set up nesting. I have a feeling they're under the overhang of Square Ledge, based on vocalizations. I get a shiver up my spine as I realize again how very privileged I am to be here, sharing the same air, the same space, the same time and place with these finely honed flyers, so perfectly formed for the environment they inhabit.

2:30 P.M.

I spy a large peregrine, a female I believe, and she wears a band. On close inspection it is black over green and 4 over 6.

3:15 P.M.

Even with a cool breeze coming down off the mountain, the black flies are awful. They even find their way into the inner space of my ear and buzz till I think I will go mad. I pick up a corner of my lunch napkin and poke it in one ear, jabbing around until I no longer hear that sound. I pull the end of the napkin out and, stamped into the nap, the tiniest black spot of an insect, dead on arrival, and no more buzzing. I settle in and watch as the female peregrine swoops and swings in the air again, this for the third time. Now I watch as she settles on the nest ledge, vocalizes a single-note call, and disappears within. I suspect the male is nearby and will come to her with food.

3:25 P.M.

Here he comes, banking in from the left. I watch, amazed as always, as the prey exchange occurs; a gentle landing and a carefully orchestrated exchange between the two of them mesmerizes me for the few brief seconds it takes for the handoff to occur. These parents caring for each other and for the young soon to be hatched remind me of the bond husband and wife share and how carefully the mother feeds her child. I think of Andrew and the close-knit bond between him and his mother and between them and me.

3:30 P.M.

I see the band on the female again and reconfirm that it is black over green and 4 over 6.

3:45 P.M.

No activity, but I keep watching.

4:00 P.M.

Peregrine activity at a standstill and I write to my heart's content, try to capture in words the feelings in me:

Me and the peregrines—
Way up here in the mountain
The streams run like fountains.
The bugs are bad;
Man, I feel "had."
The female, she's an adult!
The band she wears
Comes in pairs.
Many trees have fallen
This falcon family is calling
She's looking into the nest
Mothering at its best.
She gathers up the prey remains
Bones and feet of fallen birds, just not the same
When feathered and with wings to fly.
Up here the bugs are more than just a few
They're eating me, but do not kill, it's true.
Dualism in this place: one dines the other dies,
Or, is the eternal meal divine!

Up here with them, perched on this rocky pile
A place to spend a solitary reverie this long while.
A thrush calls "e o lay, lay o e." Then,
Another echoes, perfectly, a haunting beguile.
And I, a speck, that sits so humble
Amidst internal scars and memories so much a jumble.
But up here she calls, close to heaven and to me,
In the realm of sphagnum moss, bog leaf

And the holy feminine, a female peregrine
Begets life to young upon this solitary rock, her nest.

Sun

The sun is gone, slipped behind the rime
a frosted coat that mountains wear
in the darkest pockets of the year.
And, citizen scientist, part of life's complexities,
I cheer to health in nature, and realize
an endangered species of our state survives
in me.

Talons and Tarsus

Nails like fishhooks
Twin Tarsus bands
Black over green
Alpha numeric
Bands for life,
I get USFWS Wildlife Certificate.

Time

Our time together ends for now
Up here, where earth firmaments
The floating sky.

5:00 P.M.
There has been no more activity by the peregrines, so I pack out and
head down the mountain—a day full of things written and unwritten
and yet to be written . . . a story of my life yet to be lived and maybe even
a book someday. I stay wide open in mind and body now to whatever
is offered.

24

Vagueness

A moment's affliction brings forgetfulness of past delights;
when a man dies, his life is revealed. Call no man happy
before his death, for by how he ends, a man is known.
—Sirach 11:27–28

I stand still, holding my son, barely two hours old, and weep. My heart aches and my head reels from the immensity of this tiny life held between my two arms, which could almost fit in the palm of one of my hands. I almost died, yet here is fresh new life spouting from my own soul. My wife is asleep in the hospital bed and it's just me and this barely birthed new life come from me, a damaged, discarded, and discharged solider. The fog of existence clears just a bit as I touch, hold, and feel this life renewed. It's why we exist, really, to pass on the life we have in us to another . . . miracle of creation.

Does a baby give us purpose beyond the promise to our spouse, the duty to country, wounds that hurt, kill, maim? Vague feelings of nothingness, a black hole in mind and heart, fill the cracks between my joy. I'm not quite sure how I got here, what really happened back there in the desert. Was my heart the matter or was it my head that caved in? Why did it happen the way it did for me? Why can't I remember exactly how it came down? But I try: bright glare, punched in the head by rock-hard wood, brain bruised, contused not punctured; head and neck twisted and bones wrenched out of alignment; eyes jiggled in sockets like a bobble-head doll's. But it's all foggy, ghostly hosts from far away where the land is flat, dry, gritty, haunted; a peace that eludes me, one that I so desperately seek, just like the land that wounded me—a place fraught with the illusion of peace and where safety is in full retreat.

Andrew cries out and Carol wakes. I hand my son back to his mother.

I walk out of the room and into the sterile gleam of the hallways and nurses and the septic smell mixed with the covered-up odor of bedpans and bodily decay. I hate hospitals at the same time that I love them; they treat death and life and make no difference between them.

I take out my camera and walk back into Carol's room. She's awake and smiling at our son. We picked his name while he was yet unborn. Andrew is a good name (in the Bible the apostle Peter became a fisher of men, whereas Andrew became a fisher of individuals), a strong name for our little son.

It's two years later, and I want to go back and remember, reconstruct that memory of Andrew's birth. I'd ached from front to back and top to bottom, and his birth took that all away. Now it is back and I touch the jagged scar through my shirt.

I jumped out of the jeep, or was it a—what other kinds of vehicles did we have over there? I was stationed at Bahrain in Saudi but made incursions into Kuwait. I was an E4 in an E5 slot but no promotion. My best buddy was by my side. We carried guns, and I remember how hot it was, always that dry heat that cracked my lips, and any other exposed skin, wide open, like dry cold in New Hampshire when I was a kid building snow forts and playing army with sugar maple branches, sticks for guns, and the sound of our voices rapid-firing imagined bullets. "Sam down, Bobby down, Joe wounded, where's Henri?" They would writhe on the ground, dying a TV death with Joe dragging a wounded leg behind him trying to make it . . . to where? I cannot remember really where Joe was dragging himself. I was the enemy and he was dragging himself away from me or to behind the fort's pushed-up snow wall, packed hard as ice. We laughed and moaned and pretended in our innocence that nothing like this would ever happen to us in real life.

I was deployed with a bad heart. I still ask, even now, after the fact, why the docs would do that to me. They said there was no time not to deploy me, although they knew I had a defect in the left part of my heart.

I was headed for Airborne School at Fort Benning and then the war and then the wound that eventually ruptured my heart—a full-fledged aneurysm. I remember being in and out of sick call, finally medevaced to the USNS *Comfort*. It was not anything like what is shown in the movies, as I remember it. I did not get medevaced for my head injury but only for my heart, although head is what got me discharged . . . or was it the heart? Or both?

I don't know why this scenario keeps playing, rewinding, and replaying in my head, but it does. I apologize for all the replays of this event, but it is just the way it is, wounds adhere the body to the time and place of the wounding, leaving the mind to wander in and out of the present, almost at will, trying so desperately to realign thoughts, feelings, and memory into a more linear sequencing of time . . . but it just never happens no matter how hard you try. The bodily pain and loss remain embedded in the time of wounding, it seems never to fast-forward to the present but always remains back there, in the past, but with the feelings, emotions, and thoughts happening right now, in the current moment.

Then the Scud hit the admin building over there and I disappeared. Life died in a Scud attack while I was being prepped for surgery over here after I finally got to Walter Reed. That's another piece of this vagueness; I was flown from the theater of war to the ship, *Comfort*, then to Germany to Andrews Air Force Base, and then sent by vehicle all the way to Portsmouth Naval Hospital in Virginia because that is what the paperwork said. I tried to tell them I was army but no one listened. Even worse, the army notified my wife and she drove overnight from New Hampshire to meet me at Walter Reed. I wonder what her face looked like when they told her I was not there. So how did the army get it right with my wife and not with me? I arrived at Portsmouth Naval Hospital and when I went to check in I told them my story and immediately was denied care or concern, was told to find my own way to Walter Reed, the navy could not help me any longer. But if I could wait a few weeks, they could possibly get the paperwork sorted out; all my records burned up, and me with them, over in Saudi, where Kuwaiti oil fields burned black in the middle of the day and where my unit was deployed into an open-air dumpsite full of toxic waste. Someone up the chain thought this was a great idea, as no one would think to attack an open disposal area. I remember the smell; I had to wear a gas mask just to walk around in there. No wonder we all came back with GWS.

How did I make it to Walter Reed? Some guy in the hospital, maybe a doctor, said he would drive me there in his car, as he needed to go to Bethesda for something or other. I am certain he was navy, not civilian but maybe navy civilian. He was civil and sympathetic. So that's how I got to Walter Reed from the Middle East. Wounded and hurting in the head, heart riddled with pain and weakened by an aneurysm ready to burst, not feeling well, and in distress, ignored, and told I was on my own—I was not going to be treated at a navy facility stateside. Being in the war, in theater, did make a difference in caring, I guess. Whether you wore blue, green, or beige camo over there, you got help. But not here, not in the states, where things like uniforms and service membership mattered more than physical condition.

Rehab was another funny business, full of the stuff that others thought was really good for you. Yeah, some good, some not so good. But Carol was there, and she made all the difference. My sister did good back in the day to introduce me to Carol St. Onge, now Carol Vallieres, both of us French, unsure if that matters or ever mattered. Carol doesn't talk much about things that went wrong because now she has Andrew and I'm glad. She was so worried about me but was always there doing what needed to be done without falling to pieces, without complaining, but just supporting me and doing what was asked.

She doesn't like to talk about those tough days now, likes to forget them, but they keep coming back in ways that I wouldn't suspect. I'm still trying to figure out why when my head caved I was not sent stateside, I was told to get back out there and join the fight. Constant headaches, those damn air raid sirens, oily smoke, all sorts of scares about bio-weapons, and that time General Schwarzkopf dropped by for lunch and asked for a map and I gave him one that I had drawn. I felt awesome for those few seconds, handing off my map to the general . . . good old Stormin' Norman. He gave some sort of talk to us while we ate. I don't even recall now what it was all about except that he used my map and how good that made me feel. That is the one clear memory I have from my time in theater.

Carol and I lived in Fayetteville, North Carolina, for a while, then moved to Fort Shafter in Hawaii. Nice gig that was. Then I got accepted to Airborne School and the war came, intruded into our lives like lava flowing down the side of that bad-ass volcano on the Big Island. I personally liked Fayetteville more than Hawaii, but that's me. Carol just would come along and not complain—well, not about the little stuff. Glad she's who she is because she helped reconstruct my life after the Scud took me out over there in the desert. How can your government, the U.S. Army, lose you in that way? How can your unit commander then declare you dead just because he couldn't find you, didn't know where you were, or didn't care enough to find out? War is a damn crazy business and then it ends. You either come home or you don't. Body bags are a fact of war, but so are those other things you come home carrying, the things that war has left you with or without—tattered emotions, missing hands, feet, legs, brain parts, heart parts, groin parts, or faces burned and blasted to the point of almost no return. And, yes, you get to carry your weapons back, along with gas masks, packs, and rucksacks. Oh yeah, and what about lung tissue . . . a big one in this war . . . full of venomous fumes of oil sands burning, or was it the raw oil? It doesn't matter; it was black, corrosive, and suffocating matter that was inhaled and implanted inside the linings of our respiratory organs, and it had consequences.

25

Red-Tails, Peregrines, and the Church

Life is not measured by the number of breaths you take, but by the moments that take your breath away.
~Author unknown

Peregrine Falcon Observation, Mary Baker Eddy Church, Manchester
8 March 2008; Snowing Moderately, Wet, Cold, 34°F

8:30 A.M.
Peregrine falcon perched atop southeast parapet.

8:45 A.M.
I observe and note a silver band on the right leg or tarsus. The left leg has a band as well. Squinting into my binoculars, I can read the band: 1807-76404; green over black, 4 over 6. This adult shows lots of horizontal barring under its wings and along its flanks, heavy spotting on the lower chest and belly with a few stray spots up toward the neck, and a nice yellow cere and eye ring with a blue-black crown—majestic!

8:58 A.M.
Peregrine shows off silver band again as it stretches its wing, then its leg, flexing its talons, golden yellow and reptilian with inky black curved nails.

9:01 A.M.

Peregrine shifts and I now see green-and-black band on left leg.

9:05 A.M.

I see both legs and both bands.

9:10 A.M.

Wow, red-tail zooms by over the top of the steeple. Gorgeous view of rusty red tail and white-as-snow under parts with barely a belly band. I watch as it flies north and circles, higher up in the sky, until it disappears above the snow line then reappears; poetry in motion, so to speak. I wonder if its mate is nearby. It is early for these raptors to be up this far north, but in a couple of weeks I should see more. Do they build nests while snow is falling? Will this one find its mate of last year or have to woo a new one? If they find each other again, will they use the same nest as last year? I feel inadequate about my knowledge of red-tailed hawks. Will I ever know enough?

. . . about them, about myself, about peregrines, God? Blue jays keep up their incessant calling, a good sign that raptors are nearby. Both the flyby of the red-tail and the presence of the perched peregrine, along with the incessant creaky call of the blue jays, sends an aliveness through me like a spark or the feel of an electric shock but calms me, too, and settles me into the contour and rhythm of snow falling, birds flying and calling, and knowing I am right where I should be despite conditions not made perfect. I look over toward the Merrimack, at its high-water level, yet there's silence in the movement way over there that calms me as the snow falls. Distance from any object makes looking at it or hearing it, or living with it, different, sometimes even indifferent. Blue jays call again like a squeaky clothesline reel, or just a memory of that squeak these days, with electric clothes dryers in almost every home, those machines that are quiet and full of static, full of the loss of sound and function that are hidden inside the big drum.

9:30 A.M.

Yes, red-tail sallies forth from under the pressing snowy clouds and circles low over the eastern horizon. I say a silent prayer and watch until I lose sight of this regal raptor called red-tailed hawk.

10:30 A.M.

I keep an eye on the lone peregrine still perched stoically on the southeast parapet of the steeple, a soldier guarding the high ground, a heavenly spirit warding off evil, a lovelorn groom looking, searching for his long-gone bride. Suddenly the peregrine flaps and glides low over the land on the opposite parapet on the northwest side.

11:00 A.M.

No action, so I take lunch out of my bag and eat. I scan the horizon in all directions but snow drops drip down the lens of my binos. Nothing is moving that I can see; peregrine still perched on the northwest parapet.

12:17 P.M.

It's cold, and the snow is still coming down. The peregrine now has a dusting of white across its head and mantel. Then another peregrine appears, apparition-like, out of nowhere and lands on the very top of the steeple. Looks to be a male in comparison to the other one's size. It flies away east, then banks south, lands, and perches again at the top of the steeple. Peregrine perched on the southwest parapet, female I ID'd by size, gets up and flies southwest, then swoops back to the northeast and perches on the northeast parapet.

12:20 P.M.

Male flies off the steeple to the south and perches on the edge of the church's roof. He is now below her. She looks down and does a slight head bob, then shakes, releasing captured snow from her feathers. The male seems unmoved and keeps still, then stretches out his left leg. He has a band—black over green, 6 over 7. Both birds are banded.

12:25 P.M.

Male flies off the church roof edge, circles, and comes back, landing on the top of the steeple. The female cocks her head upward and back but remains stationary on the southwest parapet.

12:59 P.M.

Female leaves perch and flies close to male and then returns to her perch on the parapet.

1:07 P.M.

Female calling as she turns and faces north. She stretches her leg and shows off her band.

1:11 P.M.

Two crows fly through peregrine falcon observation area.

1:15 P.M.

Female leaves perch and flies north to bridge, soars and swoops from side to side, then returns to perch on the church, this time landing on the south middle roof edge.

1:20 P.M.

She turns her head and faces north.

1:27 P.M.

She turns her entire body several times, right to left and left to right, in a few minutes' time. I wonder if she is hungry, looking for prey, or just vigilant. Her belly band appears to be a peachy color. The male remains perched on the steeple top.

1:30 P.M.

The color of the sky dims, and I wonder how much longer I will be able to see anything farther out than my arm can reach . . .

    . . . *arm reaches, IV lurches as I lie in the desert on a stretcher, waiting for the chopper to come for me. Medic comes and checks, offers me water and some shade as he bends down and lifts my head so I can drink. I look up and it is so bright that I lose sight of him, my arm, and the cup that is offered; only feel the tepid, oddly dry feel of the water touch my lips. I know it's liquid only when I swallow and my tongue disengages from the top part of my mouth, stuck there from the terrible lack of moisture. I look up and notice two large black birds soaring—real or not, I can't say. They look like vultures waiting for their next meal, for a carcass lying dead or almost dead on earth . . .*

I take one last look east, west, north, and south and suck in my breath as I watch two red-tails dance along the thermals and through the ever-increasing snowfall, tails blazing red fire through white ice. I am alive in this moment in a new way, a feeling akin to a hot wire coursing through my blood, pinging every sensory organ to the melting point. It's like a painting set to animation, a magnificent contrast moving across the landscape of my eyes, seared into my being, and now I have become a part of the canvas with them.

1:47 P.M.

Observations are over for today. I get in my car and drive home, deeply satisfied at having seen both peregrines and red-tails this day. Perhaps some divine intervention happened here at the church.

26

A Journey of My Own

Hope is the thing with feathers
That perches in the soul,
And sings the tune without the words,
And never stops at all.
~Emily Dickinson, "Hope"

Peregrine Falcon Observation, Mary
Baker Eddy Church, Manchester
17 October 2007; Clear, Cool, High 40s F

8:30 A.M.
Peregrine falcon perched atop northwest parapet.

8:45 A.M.
I immediately note the silver band encircling the right leg. I also note a band on the left leg, which I can read: 1807–76404; green over black, 4 over 6. This bird shows lots of horizontal barring under its wings and has a startling yellow cere highlighting the front of its forehead, very dark eye ring black as coal, and a dark crown, the kind of black that absorbs rather than reflects light.

8:58 A.M.
Peregrine shows off silver band again as it stretches its wing, then leg, flexing its talons.

9:00 A.M.
Peregrine shifts and I now see green-and-black band on left leg; also, chest is heavily spotted and spots extend up to neck area.

9:02 A.M.
I see both legs and both bands . . .

. . . I see both of my legs, and my hands still attached to my arms that are still joined to my shoulders. My fingers move and toes wiggle underneath the thin sheet . . .

9:13 A.M.
The peregrine disappears . . .

. . . at least I lost only parts of me, and only those parts that they could cut away and then repair. The rest just got slammed against itself. And now my head doesn't work right and the pain is constant but more like white noise reverberating in the nerves, bones, and soft muscle fibers. The wound's really all on the inside, except for the Frankenstein scar running like a spiderweb from my chest, just under my heart . . .

I look down and appreciate my hands, my arms, even my nails that keep growing even after they're cut off. How would I raise binoculars to my eyes and hold them steady without my limbs and fingers? What do people do when they lose their eyes, their eyesight? I'm wounded, but I still have body parts intact that allow me to drive, eat, dress myself, and write down notes. I often wonder what I'd do if I didn't. How different would my life be? Would I have succumbed to suicide? I guess the body, once accepting of the emotional and psychological damage, moves beyond the broken pieces and compensates with whatever is left. It moves beyond depression, suicide, death wishes, hating those who love you and want to help, knowing even they cannot repair the broken body. The world is so unaccepting, so unforgiving, of a body when it's not perfect. Even wounded people struggle to accept a deformed body. Perhaps we feel less deserving of God's grace when we have broken the very thing that he gave us in his image.

But the injury has also brought things into my life. I think more deeply now about my place in the world. I've rested my being in the invisible matrix of air where birds soar. I've found peace and freedom in their flights beyond the tug of gravity, the weightlessness of imagining, having wings and hollow bones, simply flying on currents of air, aloft on faith alone. For you can't see air but only feel its movement, be buoyed up by thermals, which birds sense not by seeing but by the radar of their finely donned feathers. As I continue to work with birds, study them, watch them, I begin to know them better and myself as well. I'm lifted outside my body and into my mind and into my deep psyche, where the birds and I become one. All I know is that birds saved me from my despair and gave me a place to come and see them when I felt I had nowhere else to turn. And they allow me to be who I am without interference, without clinical outcomes, pills, needles, diagnoses, and endless counseling sessions that sometimes have made me feel worse than before I had them.

I very much appreciated all that the docs did for me, but there comes a time when simply putting a physical body back together is really all they can do; the rest of the healing has to be up to each of us. We need to journey on our own for a while, but all in all, I thank my therapists and doctors and nurses and clinicians, for they held me together long enough for me to find the birds and recover my soul, find my new walk, and learn to be me again, but differently . . . and it's really okay.

27

Self-Authentication

*Self-authentication is the act of proving that something
is genuine or true without the use of extrinsic evidence.*
~Anonymous

The Fly Entertains the Falcon

Up on Rattlesnake Mountain
I am whole unto myself.
Once the saplings leaf out
nature will make it disappear—
the ledge, his perch, guardian of the hidden nest.
I listen; watch as a single fly, unworried,
buzzes by, comes back around as
far off raven calls, a barking groan.
I watch as the fly entertains
unbanded male, adult peregrine:
patience, persistence, tolerance—
he is and I contemplate—
is his the way to be?

~06 April '06, Rattlesnake Ledge, Rumney NH

Prominent Like a Jousting Spear

They sit round the truth
like martyred saints

the strong ship tilting
the mast snaps under
the unbearable weight
of the wind
still afloat battered and torn
military veteran separated
handicapped disabled veteran
rolled into one
health complaint mortality study
traumatic causes
environmental hazards related disorder
epidemiology, neurobehavioral, neuroendocrinology,
neurotoxicology, dermatology
and parasitology—yeah,
swallowed flies—
expected after exposure,
exposed impaired
melting liquid drips
drips; its sounds I hear
like a ringing in my ear;
something happened to me
over there—now, to stand
in the society of nowhere

Fall

The dew turns to ice
The colors of green,
Triggered by cool breezes,
Turn into many colors that
Give this season its name—
Fall, autumn; third quarter equinox.
Life's a game as I reach to catch
A leaf in my hand before it falls

To earth. I witness—
Life's dance,
Life's song,
Life's theme,
Life's moment,
And, in the fall I learn
To fall gracefully.

Eaglet Spire Rock Slide

Where granite boulders, large and gray
Meet with sandy-colored duff and where my
Story pitches camp, lays down and rests its soul;
Ringed by lichen, spruce and balsam scent the air,
Darkest green, scattered patches, living in amongst
The fallen bark of white birch trees. This contrast
Makes me think of hope, almost believe, it lives
Way up here so many feet above the forest floor,
Merging human consciousness with avian anatomy,
Hallowed hallmarks, denizens, of these abstract colored walls—
Peregrine falcons, winter wrens, black-capped chickadees to
Name a few.
I sit on mosaic rock at Painted Walls, fogged in, a summary
To a story, free of guilt, contagiously happy, thoroughly
Involved, at the beginning of the unwritten yet to come.
I think of Andrew, my son, and whisper, "You should be here,"
You, birth of my bones, born of my soul, myself infused,
The unfinished me finished in you.
Infinity-you, mine-of-forever entwined double-helixed
Genes of mine now shared with you;
Walk in the power of the spirit, enjoy your life, marry
A good wife, love the Lord your God with all your heart,
And with your hands do always what is right.

Fog

Fogged in at Painted Walls, I listen, hear—
Zurr zurr zurr zurr zrray, zurr zurr zurr zurr zrray
Black-throated blue warbler animates the unseen
And I become the air that hides us from ourselves
And separates the bird from me . . . hush, listen; you can
Almost touch it.

Before I Go Hawk Watching . . .

Before I go hawk watching I stand on the bridge awaiting our fallen hero,
Scott Diamond, New Hampshire born and bred. He came back home
to be laid to eternal rest as sugar maple leaves fall and lay gently on the
ground and hawks are moving south to warmer climes. I did not know
him, but he is my brother, standing tall for us all, a fellow countryman,
officer, soldier. He met his fate—duty, honor, service to country—in a
far-off place where the sun beat hot as Hades and the ground moved so
softly under his feet. He, a true patriot, and we welcome him home—
may he rest in peace back here where he laughed and played and now
lies slumbering under cover.

Improper Function

The problem with people is they all think they know better. Do they
know better, or do they just need to be hit in the head like me to see how
they function, or not? I didn't ask to be this way. So is everybody else
perfect and am I not? Am I to blame for my improper function or am I
the fault of another? Was I simply in the wrong place at the right time,
or vice versa? An army lieutenant caused this problem and he has the
education and training not to have caused it. As for me, I have to deal
with it. Who can make it okay? Is there a title for somebody who has
this problem—of cause and effect outside one's control? If so, what is
it? There's a VCR tape of the way this thing occurred with me and now
there's written observation and now all this documentation is getting in

the way of my proper function, they say. But who is the "they"? Reality is ugly for me and I'm hostile and upset. I could really hurt somebody or something. I feel like killing peregrine falcons! If I had a gun I'd go right now and kill the banded ones in the nest and bring the dead baby birds to them, the "they," just to make my point. I feel so small and I feel like I've been pissed on and dragged through mud. How can I help myself? I feel so low. I wish I was a yellow-spotted salamander. Nobody needs to see me, hidden and hard to find, a lowly serpent slithering underneath creation.

Sunday Morning

Mary Baker Eddy Church
Bell tolls and
Perched upon its spiral steeple,
An ornamented peak,
A lone peregrine falcon has come to feast.
I watch in fascinated wonder as the one bird
Eats the other.
"Do not ask for whom the bell tolls, it tolls for thee,"
I hear the dying bird, the prey, murmur to me.
Dualism confronts and mirrors itself;
As one gives up as the other receives,
I think of Jesus as the sacrificial lamb;
Body, blood, soul and divinity and watch
The people, Sunday's congregational flow,
Walk through the door and disappear deep into
The body of the church, womb of Mary.
They are oblivious to the falcon's habitation,
The struggle for survival, life's confrontation.
All this just above the wooden door as
Christians in their church will pray of
The word made flesh this day; of Jesus
And his death for us, hanging, nailed

To crisscrossed wooden beams.
I look again, and see a similarity, the peregrine, piercing
Through the body of its prey, impaling flesh,
With spike-like beak, nailing it to the bone.
Peregrine shudders and church bells chime,
Dispersing worshippers,
Well-adorned and in a hurry;
They do not pause to raise their eyes,
Where feathers fly then gently fall,
Now disconnected,
From God's living grace;
As twelve robins in a flock, fly on by
Happy, perhaps, they did not die.
The body, empty now, of the masses;
Tolling of the bell stops as I watch
Two well-carved halves made of wood
Click together, then a hand locks them tight;
Not to open till seven days hence if not Catholic.
Falcon preens; then scratches, rouses and decides
To utter "Yaricck," a single call
That the meal is finished and
No more feathers fall.
Its body shivers, swivels, and eyes watch
As two starlings roll on by,
But snap of bill and just-fed crop leaves them alive,
Makes me say "laissez-faire," your lucky day,
As peregrine blinks, then scratches and proceeds to preen.
And, leaves me to ponder:
One dead and one left alive . . .
Which one am I?

~26 January 2008

Essentials Distilled

Nocturnal; nighthawks in myth—
suck milk from the teats of goats; but really feed on the insects
of the fields; together with goats and sheep.
Cryptic in appearance, they blend perfectly;
And are suspected of witchery.
Easily detected, ruby-red eyes, reflecting light,
loud calls given at dusk, they inhabit desert regions,
grassland and forests, too. They occur
from sea level up to 1,300 feet.

Rock

Life on the Rock
Death on the Rock
Built on the Rock
Pieces crumble up on the Rock
Prey and predator up on the Rock
Watching you, surrender,
Each to the other, upon the Rock
Peregrine hangs;
Edges become ledges
I lose my mind—
didn't make it; my life couldn't take it
way over there in Saudi and Kuwait;
left turn complication, life's manifestation—
No time for affirmations, just confirmation
Two chicks are born;
and I remain alive on the Rock.

~4 June 2000

Old Man of Square Ledge #1
Monday, 25 April 2005

It is a long distance both to drive and walk to Old Man of Square Ledge. I hike through good, clean, deciduous woods deep in the White Mountain National Forest, go up across the boundary of intermittent streams and large brook crossings where the wild things are. Only my footprints know I pass. A large raptor flies across the cliff face, sun slipping through clouds. The ranger station weather report nailed on an outside wooden post calls for snow and rain. Make it up to Square Ledge and Old Man profile, sit still, waiting, for peregrine falcons to show. I build a hooch (a slang term for a semipermanent structure used as quarters for troops in Southeast Asia) to block wind and snow. Likely peregrines are not here. Yet this place of solitude, so dear, reminds me of my dad. If he were alive I'd be with him, his birthday today. I am at least in spirit.

Old Man of Square Ledge #2

The pair of peregrines found,
in flight and then in sight,
perched; now, flown out of sight.
To enduring health—
the peregrines, I am bound!

Manifestation of Raptor Migration

I ponder the depths of sky—
The sky over the Earth—
giving birth, marveling at their flight
Coming unseen, then, brought into focus,
they perch and they preen on the breath of the sky,
take flight and are gone by thermals and wind,
The awe as they fly overhead—
manifestation of hawk migration

Caught in the raptor of it all!
Hemisphere, atmosphere, hawks appear
Humanistic, animalistic, majestic
To see hawks appear—
the manifestation of hawk migration!

First Mourning Bird

Heard through my morning window
a blue jay come to visit me this day.
Do I know the songbird? Blue jay,
as the balance, as the one who walks in two?
Colors carried of sky and unending grace
This blue jay king, my feathered friend,
who is both savior and a fallen saint,
With flashy plumage 'n loud cries,
Its shrillness warns of impending doom
For food it needs to feed its hungry brood.
And thus paths cross, and one will live and the other fall
And I wonder, if all the beasts were gone,
would man die from great strife and loneliness
or not miss the loss at all?
Who would be to blame when no more
Blue jay sparks the air?
Would this life be the same, changed, or lost,
in some immutable game?
Who would be to blame,
if anyone at all?
I mourn to think of such a fate and dream
of wet jay feather rubbed against my eyes,
l'ossieaux bleu, who comes to me
as I sleep; carries peace and hope
on wings, subconscious dream, sublime.

Barred Owl Dream

The barred owl calls me out of bed
Its haunting voice, this is what it said—
Who cooks for you, who cooks for youuuuu.
Stillness, it remains out of sight.
A pair, I think,
Repeated choral, eerie echoes
across my evening slumber,
where not another sound, not even crickets'
chirp, chirp, chirp, of male wings strummed
together, hard, like a violin, is heard.
Owls all quiet now and dream stands still.
But wait, I see them outlined in
the silhouette of a deer, standing
in the marshes, wet and dark,
where only moonlight does reveal.
Frogs croak; I search the trees
and all I spy
in the hollow of my dream—
a tiny white birch,
no frogs attached.
All I've done is a silent pledge,
distant calling out my window;
now says I have to go
back to bed
where night-bound barred owls call me out;
Who cooks for you, who cooks for youuuuu?

Nation's Symbol on My Arm Inside the Rehabilitation Cage

Its strength surpasses mine,
my arm shivers in awe,

feeding, it engulfs each mouse,
eight in all.
Raptor encounter, calls *Aw, Aw, Aw, Aw*
First day it perched on me
As if I were the tree,
Medal of Honor, then its heart beat in me;
A true gift, a blessing from above;
Nation's symbol to cherish and to love.

Self-Portrait

Observation,
Dedication,
Obsession,
Copulation,
Inspiration,
Takes flight.
Ends of earth—
The edge,
The ledge,
Its aerie confirmation!
Science,
Biology,
Geology,
Ornithology,
Windows of opportunity!
Bird of prey,
Its plight,
Its might,
Creation,
Procreation,
Me, Dacron confirmation!

Up on the Hill
There I'll go
To watch a show

Way up here the hawks fly by
Man, so glad I didn't die.

Up on the hill today
Bald eagle, Cooper's hawk,
And sharp-shinned, too.

All up on the hill
So far away from desert's kill.

Where fliers without props fly by
And, me, so glad to be alive!

~24 September 2006

23 September 2007

Along came the merlin,
I watched it zip by,
then, American kestrel,
in its finery;
circles once, then twice,
and slips between two toppled peaks.
An hour drifts; first full day of fall.
Chickadees call, but raptors hardly at all.
I spy a single cloud, alone, beauty
floating in the wide-open sky;
a blue jay flatters, its colors dare
to match those of heaven up on high.
Autumn's colors begin to turn;

if you climb, you'll likely learn
true beauty, serenity, nourished, enriched, as I,
by things with wings that fly on by.
I, Robert C., with last name beginning V—Vallieres;
victor, victory, victim, valor, veteran, disabled vet
and yet I am alive!

Persistent Granite Cores

This lair of the peregrine, drips of serrate edges
and hard rock climbs; could hurt and kill, maim,
but brings to me a sense of quietude,
of peace, and substantiation. For having died
inside the body not of my own accord; then died again,
selfless sacrifice to falcons banded on granite cores,
up here, where mountains named White, persist,
solid, honest, shaped and formed by the Lord's own hand.
I listen to God's plan for me high up here, and know
He's still forming me, life's plan, from wounds and scars, tattered
    remains.
High up here, I lose the physicality, the downward press
of gravity; am buoyed on air, merging in its thrall;
the winged beings, beauty held aloft in slaty blue;
Angels, my peregrines; cutting the air with precision of purpose
That breathes hope for being into my life and forecasts
the resurrection of the world to come.

Strafford Hill

God has brought me here, a stray,
To country town quite far away
South of where I usually lie,
Where sleep and dreams do panoply
And note the same birds here as there

On this piece of rock so stark and bare.
Me, animate on top of Stafford Hill,
And all thanks go to God's unfailing will!

Pine Mountain

13 June 2008; Clear, Warm, 70s F

This place opens my pores and heightens my senses.
I realize as the flycatcher sings
and feeds its young
that the flycatchers have succeeded thus far
as the peregrines have not.
Black-throated blue warbler calls, zurr, zurr, zurr, zray.
I think I'll pack up and move on now, out of this sincere and
    moving place
at the edge of the earth where it loses its foothold,
jags off into the sky, and affords blessings
too many to count, and trust the peregrine
will hatch and fledge, renew itself and fledge its young.

Reverie on Pine Mountain, Upper Left Side

Up on top of Pine Mountain I sit and wait
In hopes for falcons' strong wing beats.
Getting here, the humping up, not knowing,
a bit tough, finding my way, all on my own.
Unison, unicycle, union, undivided pair;
We start alone and then conjoin, some divide, life collides;
dictionary sorts as does my eye, when together and when they're
    not.

Walk around and stretch my soul, uncrouch my legs, unfurl my
   arms,
Look down and find full foot and more of shedded snake,
long dried-up skein of skin; Pick it up and hold it lightly,
think of me and Dacron matrix, heart to mend, important bends;
somewhat like this shedded skin, but sans the snake that gave it
   form;
yet me alive in shape and size, snaked within my heart this part
   revived.
Think I'll keep it as a ruse, telling others this is my life contrived—
   Make them laugh
So I don't cry.
Me, alone on the edge of earth, no falcons here have given birth,
but skin is shed and life renewed—but whose? And, how and
   when . . .

Difference—Written While Raking Leaves

Raking is lots of work, and then bagged up leaves,
Dead and dying parts of trees;
if left alone
would disassemble and return to earth.
Break down the thing called status quo—
to be the dare that really cares.
To give thanks to God,
I've cleaned up my act.
The yard is all rid of leaves . . .
But why have I not let them go,
Die and come back to earth renewed?

   ~29 November 2004

Psalm 15:1

Lord, who may dwell in your sanctuary?
Who may live on your holy hill?

The chart, a meter, almost poetry, of those
Who lived and those who died—*Gulf War* stats
Positive Courage, Strength
Fighting someone else's war
Now fighting the war within
To date, 1,000 soldiers' lives cut short—
Others wounded but none not found; cleaner gig than the one
    before,
But still a list—casualties all.
Right or wrong; wrong to right;
Sacrifice they did—
A nation's might.
Blue jays swoop and call with delight.
Human difference, indifference; birds
Enthrall, oblivious to it all.

Into the Mighty Wind at Eaglet Spire, Franconia Notch

Into the mighty wind three-quarters up Eaglet Spire
Falcon's incubation begins
as into the mighty wind I look;
forms water in my eyes, a squint, a blink.
High above in heaven's sapphire sky
Mighty wind sends clouds swiftly by—
This pair caused me to hope, to dare
To find, discover, their nesting lair.
Thought it was above the cave on grassy ledge,
Turns out to lie across the spire's massive edge,
Just at its mighty tip; out of reach but for exposed lip,

tucked, grasping, Velcroed to the rock, nest is there.
Mind searches for mighty expletive to explain
deeply felt and fathomed nature clinging by unseen thread
those eyes affirm what words cannot; where whipped-up winds
    defy
wrong judgments, and corner sins; sing forgiveness—the falcon's
    song;
where I come to pay tribute, seek to find where I belong,
and grapple with unpredictable,
intemperate,
essence,
of singular me.

~11 April 2005

Springtime, Crawford Notch

The moon risen half an orb;
night is calling, temperatures falling.
The falcon's rock, place of nesting,
faces the cliff that nearly absorbs
the female incubating there, behind the half-out bush,
in wet, wild vertical crag. She won't soon be visible
to my naked eye; but then I spy a peregrine fly—male it must be;
ethereal beauty it imparts, appears a ghostly and
gleaming host, vague breast, head and feathered core,
shines against the darkened sphere, vacuity of endless black and
    hardened rock.
I now want less, not more, of intensity, insight
so lower the power of my zoomed-in scope.
Car headlights now affect my viewing, reflect
from far below, shine off the cliff, the home, abode
of *my* peregrine's soul. The pair remains steadfast
clinging to where they call home. Still there

but soon to disappear into nightfall's
darkening mood and overwhelming gloom.
I stay put as we fall into night with falcons and me
wondering aloud—how people with jobs, 8–5,
do what they do just to survive . . .

~21 May 2010

Heartbeats, Wing Beats

To know Franconia Notch is to be in its heart,
to be in its heart is to watch *Falco peregrinus* mate.
Hearts beat, wings beat—souls entwine.
To know Franconia Notch is to touch sublime!

On Mt. Willard

Sitting in the shade of lonely balsam fir,
I spy a pair of peregrines and hear
a single one calling for its mate.
I raise my cup of tea, cheered
to be in such rare company as
junco, flicker, and blue jay serenade,
a witness to nature's untrammeled parade.
Up here, high on distant cliff I've come,
where storm clouds brew and rain cleanses,
where sky darkens and lightens,
only to fall ill, to be sick;
consoled in heaven's solace and in beauty,
held imprisoned in myself.

Painted Walls Peregrines

Up here on the Kanc where swift rivers flow
All this nature to watch; catch the breezes as they blow
The wind beneath its wings, gives her lift off the cliff
Now the nest unattended but only for a moment
To guess the age of the young; measures success
Among this pair
The magic of this cliff, colorama, rapture of untold bliss
I watch from a distance, and count, so far a solo chick;
Only one for now as I wait to see adult come back
To feed
Unless you see what appears from seed; unless, unless
You know the seed, the seed of life that feeds the blessed
Up on this cliff reveals one eye and one beak, a tiny head
Dusted white, soft furry crown
Yet only for the moment the rain falls, frowns
The day, as the Swift River down below calls, calls, calls
These falcons to their nest and breeding success—
A single chick tucked deep within the grass—
Hidden, deep inside the stick-strewn nest
Rain starts and stops and begins to fall anew
Now under shelter I do crawl—
Army poncho—a quick install.
Weather always changing; wild days up on
These Painted Walls; the cliff holds hope of falcon
Song and spring reveals its precious cache,
A baby born on earth and stone—a manager;
Halcyon's much-awaited hatch!

28

Northern Flicker on Father's Day

The father of one who is right with God will have much joy.
He who has a wise son will be glad in him.
~Proverbs 23:24

Home Station, Hoit Road, Concord
18 June 2006; Muggy, Partly Sunny, 72°F

8:45 A.M.

Today is Father's Day. I heard the flicker calling at 6:45 a.m. but didn't get up and out until just now. Yesterday I was out at 7:00 a.m. and within fifteen minutes had flickers in and out of the nest hole about twenty feet up the white birch tree out back and watched as the adults removed fecal sacs from nest cavity—a housecleaning chore—and carried in food. I couldn't identify any of the food items but think they were insects.

It's very peaceful here, Hayward Brook gushing by. Rains here cause earth's erosion all over the state of New Hampshire. My father has passed on some few years back. I miss him so. Yet here the birds sing, stream sings, as the morning air is still and without a breeze . . .

. . . *air so still you could hear molecules of it forming and breaking apart, the slight electric charges of nitrogen, hydrogen, and oxygen coming together and breaking apart into or away from each other, giving us breathable O2. And me lying there on the stretcher, staring into the vacuum of "what's next?" Not knowing is always worse than knowing because not knowing leaves you in a place of utterness, where head games play out on the "guessing game" and you hedge your bets, try to beat the odds that it will turn out badly rather than okay. That was the game I played as I lay on that stretcher, in the hot-oven desert, not sweating, trying not to think, listening for the chopper that would ferry me away to hope, help, and the next step—onto the* Comfort. *That's all I knew, the rest I had to imagine until reality caught up with me and then I would know . . .*

9:03 A.M.
One of the adult flickers pokes its head in and out of the nest cavity.

9:04 A.M.
Male flicker exits nest cavity; so the male was in the nest and female is out foraging. Male is unbanded. He is very handsome, if birds can be described as such. I sit among a shrub hung with red berries. It's about 2–3½ feet high, and it averages two to four red berries on each stem.

9:09 A.M.
The female cries "oi, oi, oi" and lands a few feet from nest hole. She's a mature female and not banded—as with male, band would be evident on right leg. She goes into the nest hole and shortly comes back out carrying a fecal sac. She flies away from the nest hole to drop it in some far-off place so the scent of it is not near nest and will not attract predators.

9:10 A.M.
She then flies back and vocalizes before she enters nest hole and comes back out carrying remaining fecal sac. I don't see or hear male bird.

9:16 A.M.
A chipmunk, a real rusty red on its back, runs within a few feet of me. Spiders crawl on me in this small stand of forest I've come to for the moment on this calm Sunday morning, watching as the chipmunk scurries in the underbrush, safe for the moment.

9:24 A.M.
I begin to hear, faintly, the young begging from within the nest hole.

9:26 A.M.

The male arrives carrying food, enters the nest hole, and feeds the begging young.

9:27 A.M.

Female calls and flies to the nest hole carrying food. She quickly enters and exits as I see my first glimpse of a young bird—an adult in miniature!

9:28 A.M.

Female comes back, and her brood are poking their heads out of the hole. It looks like they have one body and multiple heads. They peck at her face and beak as she tries to push her way into the nest hole opening. She disappears amid this chaos and so do the young, following her and their next meal.

These observations are less than a minute apart but the privilege of this day is a blessing of the moment, even as the mosquitoes hunger for a bite of me and the forest spider crawls up its sticky web to the undercover of the maple leaf, caught in its intricate weave . . .

. . . Dacron weave, heart caught within its in between, blood crawls through its slippery side, only way I can survive . . .

9:43 A.M.

Male flicker feeds one of the young at the entrance hole and then disappears, dropping down into the hole. The male than comes back out and flies off in silence. He is quiet now but when courting and mating, he has the loudest voice.

9:57 A.M.

Male returns and goes right into the nest hole as I hear female calling softly nearby, "oi, oi, oi, oi."

9:58 A.M.

Female than comes to the nest opening and calls "oi, oi, oi" and goes into the hole and feeds. I can hear the constant, begging chirps from the young; I wonder how many? She comes back out and flies to a nearby branch.

10:00 A.M.

Last observation today and female still perched on the nearby branch. I note vocalizations from a catbird, a titmouse, and a cardinal . . .

. . . *the chopper comes from the west and south—or do I have that back-ward? I look at the lay of the land differently flat on my back; need to remap the directions according to the natural order of things, not my immediate positioning, horizontal and face up on the ground. The blades chop the air with a whirring whine, and I slip my eyes into the half-opened position to watch as it approaches and then adjust to full shuttered, with lids clamped together to stop the dust from hitting vulnerable eye tissue as it lands, my last observation prior to upload . . . and I pray to our Father in heaven:*

> *Our Father, who art in heaven, hallowed be thy name,*
> *thy kingdom come, thy will be done,*
> *on earth as it is in heaven. Give us this*
> *day our daily bread, and forgive us*
> *our trespasses, as we forgive those*
> *who trespass against us.*
> *And lead us not into temptation*
> *but deliver us from evil.*
> *For thine is the kingdom, the power,*
> *and the glory, forever and ever.*
> *Amen*

Happy Father's Day, Dad!

29

Nevermore

And the raven, never flitting, still is sitting, still is sitting
On the pallid bust of Pallas just above my chamber door;
And his eyes have all the seeming of a
demon's that is dreaming,
And the lamp-light o'er him streaming
throws his shadow on the floor;
And my soul from out that shadow
that lies floating on the floor
Shall be lifted—nevermore!
~Edgar Allen Poe, "The Raven"

Frankenstein Cliff, Crawford Notch
15 June 2010; Clear, Warm, Sunny, 70s F

11:00 A.M.

This year's nesting ledge is believed to be the aptly named "candlestick ledge," which juts out and up and looks like the wick of a candle. There are two horizontal crags, the bottom one holding a raven's nest. Tales of peregrine falcon observation are not always success stories. The two ledges and the impact of nature on them are sometimes inhospitable. I'm documenting this tale, my observation of such, and I call it dualism because nature is both kind and cruel, a life giver and a life taker. Many times I (and others from Audubon) have banded young peregrines here only to come back later to find them dead, their remains scattered about the nest site, most likely prey to a fisher cat. We sometimes go to great lengths only to come up short. We can only observe the birds, band them, and be happy that they are here. Sometimes they die anyway, but not because of us. Yet this is what the citizen scientist does, observes and writes down the tale, the story, and the documentation.

Back down in Manchester we documented the nesting and hatching success of a family of five peregrine young, banded them, and watched them as they grew and fledged. Then one got injured and ended up at a wildlife rehabilitation center.

Today is a beauty of a day, but this can all change in the blink of an eye. I watch as people hike by and wonder if they realize this. They seem unprepared, no hats, sunglasses, bug spray, or water, some with shoes not even fit for walking on flat ground. Are they the extremists, who come here unprepared, then get hurt and blame the mountain, nature in its unbiased state?

Thus far I haven't seen any peregrines. By this time of year hatching should have occurred and feeding the young should be well underway.

11:35 A.M.

I just located a dead raven at the peregrines' nesting spot, "candlestick ledge." Dualism happens; hunter and the hunted. I thought of the quote from Edgar Allen Poe's "The Raven": "Tell me what thy lordly name is on night's plutonian shore! Quoth the raven, 'Nevermore.'" I'm trying to see the raven's death as a good sign, prey for the falcons' young, perhaps, yet I don't see or hear any falcons, adults or young.

I look down at the parking lot and see a host of wildflowers and a butterfly at play among the blossoms—a large yellow-and-black one, a tiger swallowtail, I think. Then I look more closely through my binos and record a clouded sulfur and a skipper.

My thoughts wander to John James Audubon and his painting of a pair of peregrines. In it he emphasized the prey-predator relationship: the hunter and the hunted, the killer with his kill; the casualty of the battle; dualism in painting and in practice. These are the challenges raptors, ravens, and we ourselves face, dangers that we are drawn to in nature—out of necessity, desire, or curiosity—but don't notice really because we must come here. No humans, outside of hikers, hunters, climbers, and field biologists, know this, I think. Birds just act out of need, not desire or curiosity, so it's bit different for them than for us. But the outcome can be quite similar, always a winner and a loser when the hunt is over and the battle completed.

My eyes have seen the glory, yet in an unfruited manner! Of course, I am in the mountains and not on a fertile plain! Once, on one of my previous visits, I showed a German couple these falcons, and now I hear only silence. Still, this gives life its purpose and pause—time and what happened before and what's not happening now. I understand life better when it slows down and I can pause to define its purpose for me.

This day brings no sign of what once was a nesting pair of peregrine falcons. To find them I must concentrate on watching their habitat, mountainous cliffs, and the face of the earth. There is good in what I do. Even when the peregrines do not show, are not here, I get to share my falcon tales.

I often think of what the Peregrine Fund, a group dedicated to the conservation of the peregrine's habitat, would think of the work I do. This is a sum fraction of the whole! I should send them a copy of my notes and tales. Do they even know what we do up here in New Hampshire for our raptors? I will ask New Hampshire Audubon's raptor biologist, Chris Martin, about this.

I can see flowers in the meadow down below: golden daisies (black-eyed Susans), yellow goatsbeard, orange hawkweed, yarrow, ragweed, and eastern starflower, to name just a few.

I have been watching today for four hours and no peregrines have been present. It's close to the time when I must move on, pack out, and hump back down the trail. The absence of falcons indicates that we have a failed nest attempt. This is unfortunate, but they were here.

On my way down, I meet a man named Josh Nimon from Indiana, an interesting character who's traveling the States. He tells me about Falcon

Cam in Wabash, Minnesota (where you can watch live-streaming images of falcons on your computer), and about falcons nesting in Indianapolis. He says that they have been coming back there for seven years. Sounds like what we do here in New Hampshire. It's always nice to make these connections.

30

War and Effects

And I saw Heaven opened and behold, a white horse,
and he who sat upon it is called trustworthy and true,
and in righteousness he judges and he makes war.
~Revelation 19:11

Going through a box of my old college papers, I found this essay:

"Greater love has no man than this, that a man lay down his life for his friends" (John 15:13). I start this paper with this quote from the Gospel according to John. This sets the context for my ethical discussion about the effects of war on an individual and how filtering this experience through the lens of being deployed with a major medical issue—a diagnosed aneurysm in the left ventricle of his heart—determines health outcomes after the fact.

Physicians knowingly and under stress-filled conditions sent a soldier into battle who had been diagnosed with a heart condition. Knowing this, it begs the question of whether or not the rights of an individual soldier are respected with dignity and with proper respect from the army in such a circumstance.

I am that solider deployed in a hurry and under ad hoc circumstances during Desert Shield/Desert Storm. I was in the first wave of soldiers deployed to Saudi Arabia with the 175th Army Engineers. I came back more injured that when I left—not only did my heart blow up while there, but I also sustained a traumatic head injury from which I still suffer.

In researching a way forward with addressing this issue, I looked to a relationship between my faith and my patriotism in trying to find a basic humanity within the army. Peter Henriot, editor of *Social Catholic Teaching*, says, "Dignity depends on freedom to obey one's conscience." I am uncertain who owned my conscience when I was a soldier. Being in the army required a state of absolute command and control. The body politic of a military force is maintained solely through obedience of those lesser in rank to those of greater rank. I had independent control of myself that went only so far—and not far enough for me to refuse to be deployed when my country called and when I was told by my superiors in the army that I must go.

The doctors who diagnosed my heart condition also failed me in this regard but stated that the impending deployment came too quickly for them to craft an exemption, which takes time. I still wonder, if the deployment had instead been planned and not so precipitous, would they still have sent me anyway and not written a waiver? To these questions, there is no answer. The military is not a democracy even though it does in fact profess a clear role in defending that principled governmental form across the globe.

So, in complete compliance with army directives and military imperative, and shutting down any further questions I had concerning my health and readiness to fight on the field of battle, I deployed.

The rest is history, as they say, with my accident involving careless handling of material and subsequently my already weakened heart finally collapsing and the aneurysm almost bursting. It is easy now to look back and place blame on a person or set of persons, but in reality, things are just the way they are. They happen the way they happen and always have consequences for the one injured and also those around him, changes that affect everyone, with both positive and negative results.

Now, looking back through the filter of time, I ask if it was ethical for the doctors to have let me deploy, to have used the excuse of "not enough time" to not process a deferment. Ideally, and with no constraint or pressure such as a declaration of war by the president of the United States, I might have been scheduled for an operation that might or might not have ended with a medical discharge. But as it was, rapid deployment was the determining factor. We were a nation at war, and the military was under pressure to prepare its troops for mobilization overseas. Collective and individual adrenaline was flowing, orders were being cut, and military personnel were ordered to be ready. In further researching the legitimacy of the decision by the doctors not to inform my command of my health issue, I have found that whatever contributes to the safety of our own troops and the successful prosecution of the war is legitimate. That is what war is about. I was ordered to go and I went—but I still wonder, what if?

It is hard for me to write this down, hard for me to accept that war treats the soldier as an expendable object, one that is human but outside the bounds of individual care and concern. While writing this, I watched a presentation by a fellow soldier who was medically evacuated like I was from the battlefield of Desert Storm. Watching him and hearing about his struggles filled my eyes with tears. He and I share the same illness, "Desert Storm Syndrome," but I have more, a head injury and compromised heart. I wonder how he is doing now, seven years removed from the war.

So, we from the Gulf War come home. Some are fine and some are not. Some, like me perhaps, should never have gone. But I, as did the others, chose to be in the army, the U.S. military, and to swear complete allegiance to our government. But does not the government also have a right, just cause, to protect us, its people, entrusted to its care? In peace-time and in wartime? But I do understand the conundrum of the soldier, of anyone in the military: that we are expendable on the field of battle. We are at once what is needed to fill the ranks and at once replaceable.

What gives me hope, and lessens my pain and confusion, is the prayer that General Norman Schwarzkopf said to inspire us before we went to battle in Desert Storm. He read the Saint Assisi prayer for peace:

Lord, make me an instrument of your peace.
Where there is hatred, let me sow love.
Where there is injury, pardon.
Where there is doubt, faith.
Where there is despair, hope.

Where there is darkness, light.
Where there is sadness, joy.
O Divine Master,
grant that I may not so much seek to be consoled, as to console;
to be understood, as to understand;
to be loved, as to love.
For it is in giving that we receive;
it is in pardoning that we are pardoned;
and it is in dying that we are born to Eternal Life.
Amen.

31

Little Round Top

*Everybody needs beauty as well as bread, places to
play in and pray in, where Nature may heal and
cheer and give strength to body and soul alike.*
~John Muir, *The Yosemite*

Little Round Top Hawk Watch near New Found Lake
*14 September 2006; Warm, Full Cloud
Cover, Light Southerly Wind, 68°F*

9:00 A.M.
Arrive and set up scope; scan horizon, then vertically straight up. No
hawks; will count per-hour intervals on the hour and half hour.

9:30 A.M.
Two Cooper's hawks soar way up high, like me; I soar with them way
up here on my own!

10:30 A.M.
One sharp-shinned hawk, small kettle of fifteen broad-wings.

11:30 A.M.
One turkey vulture.

12:30 P.M.
No hawks sighted.

1:30 P.M.
No hawks sighted.

2:30 P.M.
Four A-10s fly over, engage in mock battle just under high gray cloud cover. I see four turkeys walk through the yard of a white house clearly visible over on the hill toward Bristol.

3:30 P.M.
One turkey vulture. There's a fire over in Tilton near the water tower; smoke is dense. I hear crickets calling, spy lone hiker on Mt. Cardigan as the raven calls.

3:45 P.M.
Birded until the remote-control model airplane club started flying red birds, then packed up and moved. No more birds seen today.

3:49 P.M.
I pause in my hike down the mountain and watch a blue jay as it calls, then lands, calls again, like a beggar, again and again, persistent in its need, then flies to a valley far below. The intricate details of its plumage as it goes beyond the eye of sight shimmer like a blue diamond facet and leave memory streamers in my mind. I glance up and it looks like rain, so I pack it in and head farther down the mountain trail.

4:05 P.M.
Conditions worsen to a soupy haze, and I pass a lone hiker going up. We say nothing but just nod our heads to each other.

4:40 P.M.
I stop for a drink of water and my pen jumps out of my pants pocket and scribbles across my notebook:

> A lone blue jay.
> A lone turkey vulture.
> Alone on top of Little Round Top.
> A lone human being.

As I reach the bottom and look up—
A lone hiker.

5:00 P.M.
I sit in my car and tally species seen other than hawks: robins, northern flickers, pileated woodpeckers, downy woodpeckers, sparrow species, crows, yellow-rumped warblers, common yellowthroats, blue jays, cedar waxwings, catbirds, killdeer, solitary sandpipers, belted kingfishers, and female cardinal.

32

Dacron

Oh, good gigantic smile o' the brown old earth,
this autumn morning! How he sets his bones
to bask i' the sun, and thrusts out knees and feet
for the ripple to run over in its mirth;
listening the while, where on the heap of stones
the white breast of the sea-lark twitters sweet.
That is the doctrine, simple, ancient, true;
such is life's trial, as old earth smiles and knows.
If you loved only what were worth your love,
love were clear gain, and wholly well for you:
make the low nature better by your throes!
Give earth yourself, go up for gain above!
~Robert Browning, "Among the Rocks"

Going through a box of my medical records, I found this letter, written in 1991:

In August 1989, while stationed at Fort Shafter, Hawaii, I went to Tripler Army Medical Center for a routine physical because I was being transferred to Fort Bragg, North Carolina, and wanted to try to get into jump school when I first got to Fort Bragg. On 15 August 1989 I had a chest x-ray done, and the doctors saw something in the x-ray and proceeded to do more tests on me. After all the testing was done the doctors told me I had an aneurysm on my left subclavian artery. The doctors told me that they didn't want to fix anything that wasn't broken. The doctors said I would be fine and that I was just born that way and to go on with my life, especially when I wasn't having any symptoms that a person usually has when they have an aneurysm. The doctors cleared me and said I was physically fit for jump school. In September 1989 I was transferred from Fort Shafter, Hawaii, to Fort Bragg, North Carolina.

In September 1990 I was informed that my unit (175th Engineering Company) would be going to Saudi Arabia at the end of the month. I went to my troop medical clinic to see a doctor about my aneurysm to make sure that I was physically fit to go to Saudi Arabia. The doctor gave me a checkup, and I informed him of what I had. He said to me, "If we had more time before you go to Saudi, we could send you to Walter Reed." I was cleared to go to Saudi and on 24 September 1990 I did proceed to Saudi.

In October 1990 I was unloading wood from a vehicle in Saudi in an assembly line. The person who was passing the wood to me did not wait for me to get back into position before passing the next piece of wood, and I was struck on the left side of my head with a four-by-four piece of wood. I immediately fell to the ground and was subsequently taken to the Fifth MASH Field Hospital, where I spent the next six days. I was then sent back to my unit and given medication for my headaches, which were constant. I then found out from the doctors who were treating me in Saudi, who conferred with those at Walter Reed, that I should have been sent home and not back to my unit because of the trauma I had experienced.

In November 1990 I started to experience chest pains while I was doing PT. After a couple of weeks the chest pains were more severe, and I also had tingling and numbness in my left arm and hand. I was having these pains constantly, not just while I was doing PT. On 12 December 1990 I finally went to sick call at Dragon City, and they sent me by ambulance to the Eighty-Fifth Evac Hospital, where I saw Dr. Cohen. They took some chest x-rays of me at the Eighty-Fifth Evac Hospital and gave me some medication for the pain. The Eighty-Fifth Evac Hospital then took me to King Fahad Hospital (KFH), where the doctors there performed different tests on me. After my tests at KFH, I was taken back to the Eighty-Fifth Evac Hospital and put in a ward there awaiting transportation to the USNS *Comfort*, offshored in the Mediterranean. On the evening of 12 December 1990 I was medevaced out by chopper to the USNS *Comfort*, where I stayed for approximately four to five days. While on the *Comfort* the naval doctors performed many additional tests on me and concluded that I needed to have immediate emergency surgery to repair my left subclavian artery.

On 15 December 1990 I left the USNS *Comfort* and was taken by medevac chopper to the First Tactical Air Force Staging Area in Dhahran, awaiting transport to Landstuhl Hospital (LH) in Germany. I arrived at Landstuhl on 17 December 1990 and stayed in LH for approximately ten days. While I was there I again went through all kinds of tests and was finally sent back to the United States en route to Walter Reed Army Medical Center on 30 December 1990.

I landed at Andrews Air Force Base in Maryland, just outside Washington DC, and was told I was going next to Portsmouth Naval Hospital in the Tidewater region of Virginia. I tried to tell the people in charge that I was supposed to go to Walter Reed Army Medical Center in DC... but they would not listen and only followed what orders they had been given. The next morning, 31 December 1990, I was taken by surface transport to Portsmouth Naval Hospital in southeastern Virginia. When I got there they soon realized I was an army soldier and in the wrong hospital. Personnel at the naval hospital wanted me to wait six days before they could transfer me out to Walter Reed, but I knew I needed to get to Walter Reed as soon as possible because of my condition. I then proceeded to get a ride with another person at Portsmouth who was headed up to Walter Reed. I left Portsmouth Naval Hospital on the evening of 31 December 1990 and checked myself into Walter Reed Army Medical Center on 1 January 1991.

I was put on a general internal medicine ward at first and then referred to the Vascular Surgery Clinic, where I saw Dr. Lauer and was subsequently moved to another ward closer to the Vascular Surgery Clinic. I again went through a battery of tests, and it was finally determined that I needed surgery. On 18 January 1991 I was finally operated on.

I spent the next two days in ICU and then spent approximately eight more days in the hospital recuperating from heart surgery. I was put on convalescent leave and returned to my home in Fayetteville, North Carolina. My wife, Carol, drove me home (and was with me the entire time and was even at Walter Reed waiting for me to arrive when I was transferred down to Portsmouth). I was given Motrin and Tylenol 3 for pain when I was released from Walter Reed.

On 22 February 1991 I went back to Walter Reed for a follow-up appointment and saw a doctor at the Vascular Surgery Clinic (Dr. Lauer and Dr. Gomez were in surgery) and was put back on convalescent leave for another month. I again went back to Walter Reed on 21 March 1991 for a follow-up appointment and saw a doctor at the Vascular Surgery Clinic and was again put on another month of convalescent leave. Dr. Lauer was on leave and Dr. Gomez, I believe, was in Texas at a seminar, so I did not see them at the appointment either. I asked the doctor whom I saw questions about the Dacron they used to repair my aneurysm because I read that you can get an infection from Dacron. He explained to me that there was a chance of getting an infection from the Dacron, which would make me nondeployable and then I would most likely be medically discharged from the army; the reason given would be a disability. At this time I thought I would be getting out of the service sometime in the future with a disability. I also went and spoke with a Ms. Petty in the Physical Evaluation Board Office at Walter Reed to try to find out something about Medical Boards, etc., since no one had explained that process to me.

On 18 April 1991 I again went to Walter Reed for a follow-up appointment and saw Dr. Lauer and Dr. Gomez this time. Dr. Lauer told me at this time he was going to send me back to work with a profile and recommend on my Medical Board that I was fit for duty. I asked about what I had been told the previous month by the other doctor, and he said that the other doctor was incorrect. So at that time I thought I was going to stay in the army. I went back to work on 22 April 1991 which I realized was too soon for me because of the pain I was having and the type of operation I had gone through three months before.

Dr. Lauer asked that I come back to Walter Reed on 20 June 1991 for a follow-up appointment to see him one more time before he moved to Texas. He said that he would have my Medical Board done at that time and we would go over it on that day.

I never did meet up with Dr. Lauer on 20 June. On 19 June 1991 I received a copy of my Medical Board in the mail from Dr. Lauer, which was signed only by him. The Medical Board said I was fit for duty, which I expected because of what Dr. Lauer had told me in April.

On 20 June 1991 I went to Walter Reed for my appointment with Dr. Lauer, only to find that he was not in and that I would be meeting with another doctor. While I was waiting in the waiting room, Dr. Gomez walked by and stopped to talk with me. I told him about the Medical Board I had received the previous day in the mail from Dr. Lauer and that it said I was fit for duty. Dr. Gomez immediately said that Dr. Lauer could not say that because I was not fit for duty. He informed me that I needed to appeal the Medical Board done by Dr. Lauer.

I then went to see Ms. Petty in the Physical Evaluation Board Office at Walter Reed and told her what was going on. On 23 June I returned to Fort Bragg, North Carolina, and I proceeded with typing up my appeal and faxed the same to Ms. Petty. Ms. Petty then proceeded to send my paperwork on to the Physical Evaluation Board and on Monday, 8 July 1991, Ms. Petty telephoned me and told me that the Physical Evaluation Board said I was fit for duty. I called Dr. Gomez and told him the same. He asked me to come up to Walter Reed as soon as possible.

I was never informed at the time of my operation that the use of Dacron to repair my left subclavian artery and part of my aorta would make me unfit for military service, unfit for army duty. I was told that I would have to go through a Medical Board, but that was all I was told. For approximately five months I had been told by many different people—staff and doctors—that I was going to be medically discharged. I was staying in the army and never getting a straight answer from anybody.

It has been approximately six months since the date of my operation, and I am still experiencing a lot of pain. I was told that I would have pain for approximately a year after my operation and probably for the rest of my life. To repair my left subclavian artery the doctors had to open up my ribs and they had to remove one rib to get to the artery, which is where a lot of the pain is coming from. I also have pain along my incision. When I am outside in the heat for an extended period of time I tend to feel knotting inside my chest. I went to the shooting range with my unit in June 1991, and the next day I went to sick call and was put on quarters for two days. I should not have been sent out to the range with my unit, but my superiors read my profile wrong. It took me approximately one week to get over the pain of having to lie on my stomach and fire my weapon. I also was put on twenty-four-hour duty in July 1991 and was completely out of it for one week after that. I realized that I could not stay up for twenty-four hours and that I still needed to get proper rest.

I am also experiencing headaches at least two times a week. I am told these headaches could last for another six months or even longer. I am hoping that they will eventually go away.

Postscript: That was then and this is now; fast-forward two decades, and I am still suffering chest pain, shortness of breath, bouts of exhaustion, and headaches. What the letter above does not describe are the head and neck injuries I sustained while over in Saudi. I always wonder if the head injuries sustained in that incident contributed to the increase in headaches I had after heart surgery and still have today. It's not that my brain was damaged per se but that my brain moved around inside its outer shell like a blob of gelatin inside a jar—a slow oozing and sloshing around, banging into the more hardened membrane called the skull, causing permanent abrasions or lesions that must remain as scarring or something akin to that, as I feel the hurt just under the skin, where I cannot see it, touch it, or remedy it, only feel it. Add to that trauma Gulf War syndrome and heat stress and you get the picture of not one health condition but a multiplicity of symptoms resulting from a number of different stressors to my body. Sometimes people ask me if I would do it all over again, join up, and I must admit I hesitate in giving my response too quickly. But generally I would say yes. I loved the army and still do. I signed up and said yes, pledged to uphold what the army asked me to do. When I went to look up the Army Creed I came upon the latest version, with additional text that didn't exist when I was a soldier, but it sums up all my feelings about the army pretty well. The part I remember knowing and reciting is actually just the second stanza and was called the Warrior Ethos, but I do like this longer version better.

U.S. Soldier's Creed

I am an American Soldier.
I am a Warrior and a member of a team.
I serve the people of the United States and live the Army Values.
I will always place the mission first.
I will never accept defeat.
I will never quit.
I will never leave a fallen comrade.
I am disciplined, physically and mentally tough, trained and
    proficient in my warrior tasks and drills.
I always maintain my arms, my equipment and myself.
I am an expert and I am a professional.
I stand ready to deploy, engage, and destroy the enemies of the
    United States of America in close combat.
I am a guardian of freedom and the American way of life.
I am an American Soldier.

And, oh yeah, I had another aneurysm in August 2012, while writing the first draft of this book with my coauthor. That's a whole other book or long chapter, and I am not going to say more about that. I am almost back to square one again, but the pain of recovery is extraordinary. I fell backward into fending off bouts of depression and wondered if I could make it through this time. I feel like such a burden to all those around me. When does life stop hurting so much, punishing one's body so much, creating more work for those around you and less work for yourself? I am stationary while they are moving. I crave movement in my life but sense perhaps that I need to stand still, feel more pain, be wounded in the heart again, and keep my aching heart and head resting and processing instead of thinking and acting, to find my true destiny and purpose. I Just don't know anymore and this is where I turn to God, for in those unanswerable places is where God exists, and we must pray and have faith that it will all turn out the way it is supposed to in the end. There is no way we as mere mortals can ever figure ourselves out. Perhaps that is why I turn to birds, and now butterflies, and notice the intensity of things more acutely, like the neon, grass-green carapace of a praying mantis balanced on a bright-pink, late summer zinnia blossom just outside my kitchen window, how it is waiting, waiting, waiting, without moving, for its next victim, prey that will feed its hunger and answer its silent prayer for survival.

Some look at me and say I am courageous, that I am a hero for having just showed up in a war zone. No, it's really nothing like that. I went because I made a commitment to put on the uniform of the U.S. Army and, in doing so, pledged to defend my country. That means do what your commanders say, go to war when your president orders you to do so, go whenever and wherever he orders you to go, and do it without question. I am not sure that makes me a hero; rather, I think that makes me just another soldier, a human expendable, I guess, in the larger scheme of things, where the game of chess is played out with real pawns on a more global game board. And I am just one of the many players that governments, including mine, have set up to participate, where I become one of the many human pieces that deploy to the front lines and where outcomes are full of real damage, with real pain attached. These pieces get blown up rather than simply moved across white and black squares with it all ending with the words "check mate." Some of us fall—sent home in body bags—and some are sent home in pieces, to be dealt with according to what remains, by family who don't quite know what to do now.

Another thing that irritates and confounds me sometimes, when I let it, is all the extra and over-the-top emotional outrage over collateral damage and how there should be a war tribunal for war crimes committed on or off the battlefield. I believe war is basically immoral anyway, although God allows for a righteous war, and to say that there is such a thing as a war crime is rhetorical. War in and of itself is a crime. Not that I don't believe in defending freedoms we hold dear and helping less fortunate societies, but I think self-interest plays a heavy hand in who we protect and where we deploy to do that. As a soldier, I did not question that or any other decisions made by my command or higher authorities then. I was simply a foot soldier who did what he was instructed to do. But in every war there is always incidental take, collateral damage, and unintended consequences. No matter how much we all want it to be something other than it is, war is a dirty business in which we kill each other, no matter how much moralizing and holier-than-thou speechifying is made over this or that incident. People get killed in war, whether in planned attacks, scouting missions, or mistakes, "wrong target eliminated." Unless you have gone to war and come back with some sort of ability to reflect on its meaning, you cannot moralize it into a fairy-tale ending or one that comes out with Mr. Clean wiping it all down so there are no germs left, the battlefield sanitized and glistening white with all the blood soaked up and made pure.

I remember memorizing President Abraham Lincoln's Gettysburg Address in American history class in ninth grade, the first year I had to use English as my primary language. His assertion that blood shed by soldiers consecrated the battlefield as hallowed ground, that no words of human dedication could ever be adequate to underscore their sacrifice, rings more true to me now than it did then, as I am now tempered by the actuality of the thing and not by an imagined notion of it. Read it for yourself and decide if what he said then meets your definition of truth now:

> Four score and seven years ago our fathers brought forth on this continent a new nation, conceived in liberty, and dedicated to the proposition that all men are created equal.
>
> Now we are engaged in a great civil war, testing whether that nation, or any nation, so conceived and so dedicated, can long endure. We are met on a great battle-field of that war. We have come to dedicate a portion of that field, as a final resting place for those who here gave

their lives that that nation might live. It is altogether fitting and proper that we should do this.

But, in a larger sense, we can not dedicate, we can not consecrate, we can not hallow this ground. The brave men, living and dead, who struggled here, have consecrated it, far above our poor power to add or detract. The world will little note, nor long remember what we say here, but it can never forget what they did here. It is for us the living, rather, to be dedicated here to the unfinished work which they who fought here have thus far so nobly advanced. It is rather for us to be here dedicated to the great task remaining before us— that from these honored dead we take increased devotion to that cause for which they gave the last full measure of devotion—that we here highly resolve that these dead shall not have died in vain—that this nation, under God, shall have a new birth of freedom—and that government of the people, by the people, for the people, shall not perish from the earth.

What rings most true to me is President Lincoln's statement that "it is for us the living, rather, to be dedicated here to the unfinished work which they who fought here have thus far so nobly advanced. It is rather for us to be here dedicated to the great task remaining before us." Folks back in the day did not really have to deal with so many survivors of war with multiple missing limbs, brain trauma, and heart malfunctions. And the country was empty enough and big enough for those with trauma from the war to simply disappear, go into hiding, go west and get lost in the vastness of wilderness, or get killed on some dusty, wagon-wheel-rutted street by a sheriff or deputy, as glorified in two-penny novels of that time. It's different now because we save the body that is missing limbs, we cut open the heart and remove the swelling, replace it with synthetic material that makes you disabled, and we have a whole array of docs trying to diagnose, interpret symptoms, and render the appropriate care for each of us who comes back with interior scars that lurk where they cannot be reached or seen, where things foreboding and dark hide deep within the wilderness of the organic human body.

And here I am because technology saved me. I don't dislike or reject technology but wonder when we all reach the law of diminishing returns, when there is simply not enough of a body, a soul, a life worth living to save anymore, and then what? But the problem with that moral dilemma is, it does not include pain and suffering, either singly by the patient or collectively by those who love and care for the patient. Pain is a diffuse and individual reaction to material damage to the organic body, and I have been told that emotional pain may even be worse than physical pain. So there you have it. When is enough enough, and when should we/I press on? And what about God? Humans run afoul of humanity when they decide to play the "who lives, who dies" game. Suffering renders us human and brings us closer to God. That's all I can say—life begins and ends with God.

I stop here and think of my wife and my son. My wife is still the angel she has always been, taking care of me and the house and running off to her job. My son is off to college now and becoming his own man. I am just three weeks removed from coming out of my second open-heart surgery to repair a second aneurysm, in almost the same place as the first one. No reason to say why I had this recurrence; I just need to heal and feel better again. The pain is awful, a nightmare of déjà vu, really. And I don't feel as ready to cope emotionally as I did the first time because now I know how hard it is to heal and how long it takes. It hurts to breathe, to swallow, to blink my eyes, raise my arms, slip my feet into my slippers, button my shirt—and forget about socks and underwear. Please don't feel sorry for me, just pray for me and for all who are full of the stuff they carry on the inside and the outside, because I cannot say anymore which is worse, physical pain or emotional pain, and I have no idea what people do if they have no God to turn to in times like this. God is where all our questions end without an answer—he is the answer, we just need to be still, watch butterflies and see hummingbirds sip nectar, love our families, hug our children, and keep breathing . . . and believe.

33

One Cup of Tea

The rising sun, flickered through the bare
branches of the trees.
A few birds perched on the branches.
Free.
She sat there looking, pondering, wondering.
Her fingers, wrapped around the cinnamon
stick, stirring her tea.
She thought about her life she yearned to
free, as she raised to her lips
the cup of tea.
~Anonymous, "The Tea Cup"

Banks of the Merrimack, Concord
8 January 2010; Snow Falling, Poor
Visibility, Bitter Cold, High Teens F

11:00 A.M.
Adult bald eagle perched in deciduous tree on east side of riverbank.

11:15 A.M.
Then it flew north up the river, disappeared through the sheets of snow falling.

11:20 A.M.

I tried to walk along the railroad track but visibility almost down to zero . . . maybe thirty feet, or up to seventy feet between snowfall bursts.

12:34 P.M.

Back at truck, I took a walk out on bluff on west side of river, a noisy group of people on far, or east, shore. Bitter wind; gave up, with little chance of seeing more eagles.

Banks of the Merrimack, Concord
9 January 2010; Clear, Bitter Cold, North Wind,
Blowing Snow, Teens F with Windchill

6:45 A.M.

A continuation of yesterday's observations on the west bank of the Merrimack River. I observe red-tailed hawk perched on a small shrub close to the water's edge near the bend in the river heading south. Sun not up yet but the barely brightening sky and the slim color just starting to define the eastern horizon hold hope for a clear day.

6:52 A.M.

Large adult bald eagle flies along the east bank of the river at the bend. I can hardly write notes, my fingers are so cold. I watch as it flies north, makes two low circles, then comes back south, soaring low just above the tree line—hunger on its mind, survival its imperative as it flies just above the open water of the river now. It's so cold I stand and shiver to keep warm.

7:10 A.M.

Red-tailed hawk launches from its perch and flies north, skirting the east bank of the river. Its fiery tail is the color of

. . . rocket propulsion during liftoff or Scuds as they land and explode, tails of tracer rounds through the darkness—flickers of red and other colors, even white . . .

7:25 A.M.

Observe adult bald eagle flying along east bank just below the tree line from south to north. Same one as before and very large. Now it crosses the river and is directly overhead, maybe sixty feet above me. I am in awe and get good looks at its yellow bill and feet, power in motion. I follow it as it disappears north out of sight. I am pumped! Another single bald eagle appears, smaller than the previous one—male perhaps? I think it came from under the bridge. It flies north, upriver, and disappears from my sight. I scan river and note a goldeneye skimming just above the surface of the river. My fingers are so numb I cannot feel them; temps in the teens and nothing in between!

8:40 A.M.

A single, male red-breasted merganser flies south just above the water and lands in rapids below the falls. How can they tolerate that much cold water?

8:48 A.M.

Adult bald eagle, the larger one, flies south into my field of view toward bend in the river near the farm. The bend is commonly called Merrill Farm Bend. Eagle flies low to the river again, seeking prey, I would suppose. So far have seen eagles three times—two of the times I am certain it is the same individual, the very large bird; the other time I am uncertain but think there are two birds because I noted another eagle flying north after I had observed the larger one fly out of sight. The cold has so numbed me that my fingers and my eyes do not work together in my observations— seeing and writing down what I see. Two blue jays brighten the cold with their sky-blue backs and snowy-white bellies. They're beautiful birds but common, so we miss their beauty or get so used to it that we forget to admire their good cheer on such a cold day, or any other day . . . like we forget to love everything in our lives that we get used to.

10:25 A.M.

Back in my truck, I start the engine and crank up the heat, eat, and write:
Stand out in the cold only to shiver,

Along the west bank of the Merrimack River
The weather so cold, the river so bold
One cup of tea, please, to ward off the cold!

10:56 A.M.
Back outside, I watch as large masses of ice go floating by. I look south at a large pine and observe bald eagle adult perched with back to me, head and tail white as the fresh snow that fell and covered the ground yesterday. I watch it lift off, fly across the river, and meet up with another adult eagle, slightly smaller in size; wonder if they are a pair? This confirms that I did see two individuals before.

12:25 P.M.
I keep watching and need to move around to keep warm. Windchill is bitter and goes right through me. I now observe the two adults and an additional eagle, a subadult, perched nearby. Is this last year's young? From this pair? Bitterly cold and the wind chills me to the bone and beyond.

12:47 P.M.
Adult bald eagle flies from south to north.

12:55 P.M.
Adult bald eagle leaves perch and flies along east side of the river just above tree line, skirting past pines, and disappears south. I get in truck and cross over the river to the east side.

1:03 P.M.
Went hiking on east side of the river behind the Concord Monitor building, stopped and checked various lookover areas, walked along the bluff going north. Great views of west bank and both north and south up and down the river.

1:30 P.M.
Back in my truck feeling satisfied that I have done enough for today; it's just too frigid cold, and with the biting wind, I can't stand being outside any longer. I rub my hands together, cold and stiff . . .

... stiff as a corpse, all dead and cold and white as ice ... not able to be warmed by a single cup of tea ... can't even grab the cup offered me. I like coffee better than tea ... hot drink in the desert but I feel so cold. A shadow passes overhead—vulture or chopper far away from home? My fingers stiff and I drop the cup of tea, watering the desert. Is it a bird or chopper shadowing me, passing over me, coming for me—dead or alive? The mind does funny things to you when you're lying in the desert. Wavy lines of heat blur your vision, then you blink and clear your sight, wake up, and discover it was all a dream, pointless, imaginary unreality, and you wonder why it is so hot and you feel so cold. Did Jesus feel cold when he died on the cross?

I quickly tally numbers and leave for home a few miles away, thinking just of being warm inside and outside, my fingers entwined around a cup of hot tea.

34

Cages

BY JACQUELYN M. HOWARD

I know what the caged bird feels.
Ah me, when the sun is bright on the upland slopes,
when the wind blows soft through the springing grass
and the river floats like a sheet of glass,
when the first bird sings and the first bud ops,
and the faint perfume from its chalice steals.
I know what the caged bird feels.
I know why the caged bird beats his wing
till its blood is red on the cruel bars,
for he must fly back to his perch and cling
when he fain would be on the bow aswing.
And the blood still throbs in the old, old scars
and they pulse again with a keener sting.
I know why he beats his wing.
I know why the caged bird sings.
Ah, me, when its wings are bruised and its bosom sore.
It beats its bars and would be free.
It's not a carol of joy or glee,
but a prayer that it sends from its heart's deep core,
a plea that upward to heaven it flings.
I know why the caged bird sings.
~Paul Lawrence Dubar, "Sympathy"

Tuesday, 13 March 2012

10:00 A.M.

I meet Robert at the New Hampshire Audubon Society headquarters at 84 Silk Farm Road in Concord. The day is surprisingly pleasant, around 60°F with a cool, 10 mph wind from the northwest. The sky is the type that makes you float upward, feet unhinging from the ground. The longer you stare, head craned perpendicular to your shoulders, the less you are substance and the more you become the wind, the blue and white matter of heaven, floating in antigravity.

And then Robert spots it, the first broad-winged hawk of the season. Robert's yelp brings me back inside my own skin and hands; my feet grid the ground. He hands me the binoculars so I can see what he sees, a small dark object tucked just beneath the large white billowy cloud to the east, soaring against blue so intense that it reminds me of a Maxfield Parrish painting.

Such is time spent with Robert, and I am lucky enough to have been invited to visit him on a day when he will be working in the cages, caring for the large birds of prey that are injured in some way or another and will never go wild again.

10:15 A.M.

Robert directs me inside the building, and we walk to the back, then turn right and go through a smallish door where the food and some other miscellaneous supplies are kept. He explains that we are going to enter the cage of the eagle but, before that, he will open the door to the owl cage.

I am instructed to stay behind and let him enter first, as the birds know him. "Wait till I call you and then come in quietly," he tells me.

10:18 A.M.

Robert picks up a very large and sturdy glove made of leather and suede and long enough to extend up to his elbow. He puts it on his left hand.

We proceed inside the outer walkway of the series of four cages, each with its own entrance door that is locked. Robert proceeds to the second cage door, talks softly as he unlocks it, and then enters and closes it behind him. I hear him make a clicking sound, and he then sticks his hand out the door and waves me in. The square cage is darkish and made of a chicken-wire-like material. It opens to the outside, but some sort of tarps or coverings are thrown over the roof.

I wonder if this is Robert's lair, his life now feeling like a cage, living in a slightly darkened, never completely bright space, gently proceeding onward and looking for the injured . . . in himself and in the birds he's hoping to rehabilitate. Cages are made to keep some things in and to keep other things out. Does he ever wonder if there is a way out, a way to the bright light? And if so, what might it lead to?

We spend approximately ten minutes with an owl who lives here by himself, a beautiful, mournful-eyed barred owl missing part if its left wing. It was found originally by a trucker way up north on the side of Interstate 93. It probably ran into a car or a truck and just lay there dying until it was rescued and brought here for rehabilitation. It's feeding time, so Robert lays a dead mouse on the stump in the middle of the cage and keeps calling the owl by making a clicking noise that mimics the sound the owl makes just before a kill. He backs off a bit and keeps up the clicking. The owl is tucked away up in the far corner of the cage and stares down at us. He looks toward Robert and then at the mouse but makes no move to come down.

Again, I wonder about Robert and his work in the cages, rehabbing birds. He spends hours here, feeding them, cleaning their cages, "speaking" with them, encouraging them to come and eat. He relates to them, one wounded soul to another, each in their cages—one within a physical boundary, the other behind an emotional and psychological barrier. I do not know Robert well enough to ask if he feels himself imprisoned in a cage, the body acting as a jailhouse to his deeper, wounded self that lies invisible and unnoticed, surfaced by a body that appears intact and unblemished, a hidden potential not marred by a missing part. I wonder if all his conflicting feelings are like an unexploded booby trap waiting for the trip wire to be breached . . .

10:30 A.M.

I watch as Robert carefully backs out the door of the cage, step by careful step, as if he's moving through water, always keeping eye contact with the bird. The owl stares back at him. It almost seems like they are stalking each other. As the door closes, I see the owl swoop down, land on the stump, and swallow the mouse. These cages keep injured birds safe and alive, well fed and watched over by Robert.

We precede to the last cage, where a majestic bald eagle sits, perched high on a fat stick wedged crosswise from left to right. Robert tells me about this bird, an adult female with a broken wing and a hole through her chest. She had been shot and then fell to the ground, breaking her wing. He tells me this is his favorite bird to work with here. He loves the eagle and admires how big and majestic she is. She has been here the longest of all the current birds, and he has been taking care of her for six months now. She may soon move to a rehab facility that does educational programs with schools. "I will be sad to see her go," he says.

He unlocks the small door and walks in, closing me outside it. I hear a high-pitched chirping sound and then a response. I cannot tell Robert's call from the real thing! When he signals me to come in, I enter and close the small door tightly behind me. I am in the cage with Robert, the injured bird, and more dead mice.

My heart breaks to see such a large bird restricted to such a small space and with such limited opportunities to expand its wings. When I mention this to Robert, he tells me that she couldn't survive in the wild. With only one good wing, she would fall to the ground. He says this bird is lucky that the shot went right through her and did not pierce her heart.

But she doesn't seem lucky to me, this bird who will not mate ever again, never soar over ocean and mountains, never rear young, teach them how to fly and catch fish, and ultimately watch as they leave the nest. I can't help but feel sad for such a being as this—caged, limited by her injuries, and now being fed instead of feeding herself.

I think of Robert's heart in a cage, his brain in a cage, his body in a cage, and this eagle exploding out of his chest, freeing them both. Robert has found his way out by coming in, and as he tends the wounds of these powerful birds, he tends his own wounds, exhumes his essential nature inside these cages, making life work for a broken-winged bird in the same way he is trying to make his own life work, this disabled vet with a half-rebuilt heart and a head addled in war by a stupid act of carelessness that, in the blink of an eye, turned a career soldier into a manila folder stamped "discharged disabled."

Robert and I stay in this cage about twenty minutes. He even leaves me in there by myself when he goes out and comes back in with a broom and a dustpan, beginning to sweep up the twigs and leaves and bird droppings and carefully toss them in a metal bin with a lid. He methodically sweeps the entire cage in about ten minutes.

The act of sweeping an enclosed space, cleaning it up, even the dark corners, is therapy for the soul, a physical movement, an act, a catalyst perhaps for a deeper cleansing going on inside of Robert. He is focused on the task at hand, with the eagle and me watching him, all of us inside the rehab cage. He is focused on the care he's giving, on the bird's salvation, and on my observation.

Robert turns to me and breaks my reverie, saying, "Cages can both free you and capture you. They can offer you sanctuary and set your spirit free, or they can be barricades between you and yourself, and what you most want to do with your life. I look at this eagle. She doesn't really know what happened to her except she experienced pain and could not fly. Does she know she was brought here for her own protection? Or that otherwise she would have died?" He shuffles his hat back and forth on his head, settles it back in place, cocking it slightly back so his eyes are visible from underneath the cap's bill as he goes on talking. "Her cage protects her from her enemies and the elements, which would have killed her, but why do we protect her and keep her alive? I wonder for whose benefit, hers or ours?" He smiles and holds out his arm to her, calling her. She flaps down and lands awkwardly on his leather-gloved arm. He feeds her a treat, a dead mouse, head first, and she gulps it down, the tail hanging from her fully clenched beak as she flaps lopsidedly back up onto her perch. "I feel sad for her sometimes, but then I think of the joy she brings when she lands on my arm, takes mice from my hand. Giving happiness to so many visitors, I guess, justifies our keeping her in this cage. And this rehab center has given her a new life, a new way of being, living her life differently than before—sort of like me after my life changed in Saudi." He sighs. "My cage is my own attitude about how people treat me and how I am tagged for the rest of my life as disabled. That's my cage and inside it are held my wounds—invisible but real, however unseen or hidden. It's simply my cross to bear. But I am not missing pieces per se, just missing 'normal'—having Dacron patching my heart, my skull intact but the circuitry misfiring inside it, the vertebra in my neck and back twisted wrong, and a big zag of a scar running like a shoulder harness up and over my left shoulder and under my arm."

As he talks, Robert keeps up a methodical sweeping of the floor and looking up at the eagle, smiling. I almost think I see the eagle smile back, but that can't be true. It's strange, the eagle watches over Robert as if she were the nurse tending her patient, instead of him tending her as if she were his sole concern. Looking at the two of them, I feel as if I am in an unwritten play being acted out ad hoc right before me but without a script, a subtle energy flowing between these two beings captured and held within this chicken-wire frame, half inside and half outside, half exposed to the elements and half protected from them, the two of them wounded, caring, sharing a secret unfathomable to me, each moving to an internal rhythm of his or her own making yet merging in some place within that I cannot see.

I stand here, lost in my reverie, for who knows how long, when Robert stops sweeping. He touches my elbow and says, "Ready to go?"

But I don't feel ready to leave this space, this cage full of life and catharsis, understanding and unspoken camaraderie, almost mystical happenings . . . and all within an enclosure that excludes the world's dangers and only lets in the safety, a place of redemption for both Robert and the eagle.

I turn to him and say slowly, "Yes, I hate to go, but I guess it's time to leave here." He gathers his broom and dustpan, holds open the door to the cage, and lets me out. The veiled trance I've been in breaks immediately, and I hear the hushed voices of a group in the next cage, a small group of Girl Scouts with their Audubon guide, see the bright glare of sun glinting off shiny white birch bark, hear the bark of a dog outside. I watch as Robert backs out, slides the key in the lock, and clicks it to the right. I follow him into the small room that holds the bird supplies and equipment, watch as he slips the oversized glove down his arm and off his hand and places it back on the shelf where he found it.

Then he says, "Let's go outside to the picnic table and eat lunch."

I give a silent nod and follow him down the narrow hallway and out the side door. I'm hit by a cool north wind, a splash in my face that wakes me up and jostles me back into ordinary life, real life. But I wonder which life is more real—the one inside that cage or outside that cage? Inside, it felt safe, unconditional, validating, confident, known, and familiar. It was protective of my body, no wind bashing against exposed skin, no glare squinting my eyes and causing creases, no need to hold down the dashing about of my hair, and no worrying about what needed to be done or undone.

The cage gave me a sense of safety and reminded me to consider the alternative, that this eagle could be lying, splattered, dead somewhere instead of being here, in the cage, cared for by her soul mate, Robert . . . as if the bird had his heart and he hers. I smile over at Robert. The answer is simple: Robert caring for just one being, his eagle, with whom he shares the ultimate secret. Authenticity is what cages are all about. The injured beings rehabbed in them can be who they are. The cages just give them hope of recuperation and regenerative grace, a respite from judgment and interpretation and interrupted lives: in a word, redemption. Here all that is demanded is that the eagle eats, sleeps, digests, and stretches her wings. Robert shows up to ensure that this measure of life happens. The eagle depends on Robert, and Robert depends on the eagle. Healing happens inside the cage; just because we on the outside of this miracle cannot comprehend it does not mean it does not exist. The eagle validates Robert, her eyes free of criticism or question, as if imparting to him, "It is what it is"—the very root of acceptance. And isn't that the most basic ingredient in healing?

Robert and his birds are extraordinary beings, captured prey, but in different ways, free to carry on their lives inside cages, invisible and visible, understanding that healing happens inside and outside of a person, and especially outside of clinical diagnoses and the branding with the names of illnesses too cumbersome to fit inside cages that contain spirits joined in a higher coupling. As Robert says to me now across the table, "Doctors need to write more prescriptions to go bird-watching than for pills. People need to stop looking to pharmacies for help or to small amber bottles of meds that can make you worse instead of better. . . . Just ask the eagle."

And then Robert bites into his sandwich and takes a drink from his water bottle as if nothing profound has happened here, as if life has walked him down a different path, a road less traveled, that reveals a truth as simple, accessible, and restorative as . . . an injured eagle in a cage watching as he shares time and place with her in a confined space half open to the outside world and half protected from it.

35

Wings Shift, Revealing Creation

Then God raised His arm and He waved His hand,
Over the sea and over the land,
And He said, "Bring forth. Bring forth."
And quicker than God could drop His hand,
Fishes and fowls
And beasts and birds
Swam the rivers and the seas,
Roamed the forests and the woods,
And split the air with their wings.
And God said, "That's good!"
~James Weldon Johnson, "The Creation"

Painted Walls Peregrine Falcon Observation
7 June 2007; Mostly Cloudy, Breezy, 60s F

9:40 A.M.
Adult on nest; wings shift; something under it is moving. Moments later adult gets up and walks off nest and flies away, revealing creation and a confirmation of the birth of a young falcon. The chick looks to be eight to fourteen days old. I am here as witness to this new life!

9:54 A.M.
Moments later the adult flies back and lands in a tree near the nest ledge; looks to be a female but at this distance cannot be sure.

10:17 A.M.

The peregrine remains perched in the small sapling near nest ledge. I determine that this is a female and watch as she preens.

10:30 A.M.

She flies, leaving nest and young unattended. I wonder where her mate is.

10:40 A.M.

Falcon chick appears for only a brief moment, just revealing an eye, crown, and beak above the twigs and grassy edges of the nest; now lowers head and is hidden again.

10:59 A.M.

It's windy and the rain starts so I drape my poncho over some low-hanging branches of a young maple sapling. Temperature drops and cloud cover is now complete. I watch in relative dryness as the female returns to the nest ledge and perches near the nest, which is half hidden from my view.

11:01 A.M.

I observe a second peregrine, the male, come flying in and land on the ledge, prey squeezed in his talons. The female, already perched, watches, perhaps anticipating food for her young. Size does matter when ID'ing peregrines and other birds of prey—the female tends to be larger and the male much smaller in stature!

I observe a stationary prey exchange. She takes the prey offering from the male, then goes to the nest, circles it once, and drops the prey into the nest. She then flies off. Still only one chick visible thus far. I see the chick picking at the prey, but it stays mostly hidden down in the nest.

11:20 A.M.

She's back at the ledge, perched in the small sapling nearby.

11:28 A.M.

Now she is back on the nest brooding her single chick . . .

. . . only a single young, my son, Andrew. A dream come true, light of my life, perched on my wife's lap, wrapped in a blanket that almost covers his

face. She gets up and nestles him just so in the crook of her right arm. She walks toward the kitchen, comes back seconds later with his bottle, sits back down on the couch, and feeds him . . .

11:38 A.M.
She's off the nest and flies up, circles twice, then comes back and lands in the small sapling at the nest ledge. High winds pick up.

11:54 A.M.
She hops from one branch to another, paying close attention to the nest and the chick huddled there. Off to the north I see showers approaching.

12:07 P.M.
Female remains perched. It begins to rain.

12:15 P.M.
Rains heavily. I decide to pack out and break down my poncho tent. I leave, knowing creation begets creation, and this pair has successfully hatched at least one young. Life-giving rain falls, and winds make the air fresh; all's right in God's heaven! I am truly blessed and privileged to be here and to meet the peregrines on their own terms.

36

Merrill Park

*I want to fly where no seagull has flown before. I
want to know what there is to know about life!*
~Richard Bach, *Jonathan Livingston Seagull*

Merrill Park, Concord
8 March 2006; Dense Clouds, Cold, 38°F

11:30 A.M.
First species I see is a flock of forty to fifty red-winged blackbirds.

11:45 A.M.
Walk farther along the open field and count fifteen crows and twelve
Canada geese in farm field.

12:10 P.M.
Watch as five more Canada geese fly and land in the field. They come
in with landing gear down like a helicopter, and their props, wings,
hung outward, to break the landing, act as a drag on the air pushing up
against them. But they land gracefully and noiselessly, no scarfing up
dust or snow. When they open their maws, they're mouths for eating
and sustaining life, not a portal, a way in or out, for an injured soldier,
a life hung in the balance.

12:15 P.M.
I set up my scope and scan along the edges of the field and the far tree
line. Spot a large stick nest in a white pine tree southeast of the fields

near the old white farmhouse. I'm set up at a No Trespassing sign, look-ing northeast; good perspective but a very great distance from the nest. A good discovery but wish I were closer in.

12:19 P.M.
Two mallards fly into the field and land near the gaggle of geese; the geese ensure that the mallards do not stay too near, chase them off their territory.

12:23 P.M.
I look overhead just in time to count eleven turkey vultures flying by. They are early returning migrants to this part of their summer range.

12:31 P.M.
Five gull species fly in—black wing tips. Are they ring-bills or herrings? Crows calling, geese honking, many more crows, with some pigeons, fly-ing and landing. Seven more mallards fly in; one of them looks different but I can't identify the species, think it may be a blended mallard—part black duck and part mallard. Eight pigeons put down in the field. From my vantage point I see many, many bare tree branches and possible perches, and I see a bird silhouette but cannot determine species. It could be a raptor by its size and shape.

12:37 P.M.
Blustery winds kick up. Pigeons, gulls, crows, and ducks fly away toward the river, and the geese become restless and start moving around and honking.

12:42 P.M.
A lone robin lands along the roadside. I want to see a red-tailed hawk but only the more common, field species are here—robins, ducks, geese, crows, turkey vultures, and culls. I try using my scope but too windy. It won't steady, so I just use binos but not as powerful . . .

. . . the x-ray film showed in fine, high-definition detail the bulge in my heart. It took what was invisibly inside of me and made it visible; let me see it close up even though it was deeply buried inside my chest cavity . . . a powerful image of a weakened structure—me from the inside out . . .

1:52 P.M.

Finally I see a red-tail! It is way up in the sky to the northwest, gliding over the Exit 16 sign on the highway. I follow it as it soars south to Eastman Cemetery. There it puts down in a large white pine tree, then rises again and soars northwest along the far tree line until I lose sight of it as it disappears over the roof of the Eastman School. The nest I spied earlier in the large white pine near the old white farmhouse could be its nest. I wonder if the red-tails will use it this year. Or will they use the nest I just found in the white pine near the cemetery? I will note both locations and keep checking them for nesting activity as the season progresses.

2:10 P.M.

I see a red-tail rise up from an unseen perch and then I lose it. Is this the same one I have seen or is this another, possibly the mate?

2:31 P.M.

I scan the field and the tree line, check out the horizon to the south and east, and finally look straight up and see two red-tails up and soaring, my heart soaring with them—YES! I watch as a courtship flight occurs. I wonder if incubation has started and if an egg is already in the nest? Pretty certain they're using the nest in the white pine near the cemetery. I lose sight of them again as they swoop low behind the row of trees.

2:38 P.M.

I search the sky and horizon over the trees but don't see the red-tails again. I count seventy-five to one hundred Canada geese, fifty ducks—most, if not all, mallards—and many crows and now have finally ID'd the gulls as ring-bills. I watch as they take off in a group and spiral ever upward, almost into the clouds, a sprinkling of salt and pepper against a gray sky. What seems to matter to them most is that they stay in their group and fly together as high as they can reach. I almost can feel what that is like . . .

   . . . *as I am airlifted out of the desert in the chopper, riding through the air to be deposited on water supporting a ship, a floating hospital, a sick bay for those who couldn't make it home any other way. My group is now without*

me and me without them. Time for regrouping, but I'm down for the count,
counted among the casualties of war . . .

4:00 P.M.

I'm cold. It's starting to get a bit dark, and so I call it a day, happy that I
was able to confirm the presence of a red-tailed hawk pair!

37

Larry Pelland's Story about Me

There's a victory and defeat—the first and best of victories,
the lowest and worst of defeats—which each man gains
or sustains at the hands not of another, but of himself.
~Plato, *Laws*

Come Fly with Me
. . . Through Your High-Powered Binoculars!

By Larry Pelland, *Weirs Times*, 15 October
2009. Reprinted with permission.

I recently experienced the thrill of a lifetime, as I stood in the corner of
the mighty resident Bald Eagle's "mew" (cage) at the Audubon Center in Concord, New Hampshire, observing and enthralled, as Robert
Vallieres, Hawk Expert, fed this magnificent bird of prey an entrée of
Atlantic salmon, one of its favored meals.

This majestic bird has a wing span of six feet, and weighs 8.6 pounds,
a perfect weight for an adult male eagle. On average, it takes Robert
anywhere from twenty to forty-five minutes to feed him, depending how
hungry the eagle is from day to day. After finishing his meal, the eagle
ascends to his perch in the "mew," where he reigns supreme.

How did I formally get introduced to "Hawk Watching"? Joe Quinn,
a resident of Havenwood–Heritage Heights Retirement Community in
Concord, New Hampshire, a very knowledgeable person in the pastime
of bird watching, took my wife, Rita, and I to the Carter Hill Orchards

Observation Platform in Concord, where he introduced us to the thrill of seeing these magnificent birds of prey in flight, through our high powered binoculars. It was an awesome sight to behold! Carter Hill Orchards are to be commended for their generosity and community spirit in funding the Observation Platform that is open to the general public. As Joe Quinn put it, "The more sets of eyes looking through binoculars, the better chance you'll have of seeing hawks."

On many a day you will find Robert Vallieres on the observation platform, welcoming and instructing newcomers how to best see the hawks in flight. He keeps a daily log on the type of raptors spotted and loves to interact with visitors, whether they are first timers or seasoned veterans in hawk watching.

Robert was first introduced to hawk watching some eighteen years ago while on a tour called "Birds of the North Country." From that moment on it changed his life forever and helped him to get on with his life. Chris Martin, Senior Biologist of the Conservation Department at the Audubon Center, had a huge influence on Robert's bird watching career. Today, Robert is recognized as a Raptor Hawk Expert. He is honored and respected as the "Ambassador of Falcons," "Steward of Falcons," and "Falcon Biologist." A master at his craft, Robert has dedicated his life to bird watching and rehabilitation. He is their guardian, protector, and crusader for their very existence. Each year Robert, a New Hampshire Audubon seasonal biologist/interpreter, documents hourly weather data and counts and identifies all of the raptors that pass by the mountains near Carter Hill Orchards. Visitors with a full-color key chart can identify the various raptors of New England. The best days for viewing hawks are warm and sunny, with winds from the northwest, especially during the month of September. A database administered by the Hawk Migration Association of North America (HMANA) is shared by biologists and with visitors and helps them to view and identify raptors.

Prior to his introduction to the NH Audubon Center and Raptor Hawks, Robert served with honor, valor, and distinction with the 175th Army Engineers out of Fort Bragg, N.C., part of the 18th Airborne Corps, in Iraq during Operation Desert Shield (Storm). He held the rank of E4, acting in an E5 position. While on duty, he sustained a severe head injury and returned to the United States for extensive medical treatment. Today, he is a productive member of society and his contributions are numerous. The joys of his life are his wife and son. "They are a gift to me," he commented. Thank you for your service to our country, Robert. You in return are our gift.

Robert is often called upon to rescue birds of prey, always rising to the challenge under unusual circumstances. Point in case, he rescued a hawk stuck in a chimney in a residential home. He is always eager to give talks on bird watching, and his enthusiasm shines forth brightly during his presentations.

Some of Robert Vallieres's interesting observations . . .

"We do not name the birds. They are not our pets."

"The peregrine falcon lives today because somebody took care of it and reintroduced it into the world."

"We discovered marlin falcons nesting in Concord off of Stone Street, originating from the North Country."

"Eagles and other birds of prey have a natural protection from the sun in the form of oil inside their eyes. The oil filters out the UV rays and prevents damage from occurring, thus enhancing the bird's vision."

"The eagles can turn their heads 210 degrees, while the owls can turn their heads 280 degrees."

"Raptors are a symbol of power, health, and vitality."

There are many terrific volunteers who give of their time and talents at the Audubon Center. Marlene Freidrich, staff naturalist, is one of those stalwarts who loves her work. On any given day you will see her at work, often displaying a barred owl on her gauntlet, showcasing it to visitors, young and old alike. Children especially love to ask her interesting questions about these fascinating birds of prey.

Birds of prey, better known as raptors, include hawks, kites, eagles, falcons, and owls. They hunt other animals for food. All have strong claws for grasping prey and bills designed for ripping flesh. Owls hunt primarily at night, so they are called nocturnal raptors. The others hunt primarily during the day and are called diurnal raptors. Certain species, such as the peregrine falcon, were pushed to the brink of extinction by the use of a chemical called DDT. A major effort by conservationists, plus protective laws, helped the peregrine falcon to recover.

The Audubon Center offers great programs, including live animal presentations, arts and nature, photography, birds of prey featuring a live bald eagle, outdoor adventures, and wonderful family programs that are free. If you haven't visited the Audubon Center of NH, located on Silk Farm Road in Concord, you really need to check them out. After your first visit, you'll be enthralled, wanting to return time and time again. It's an educational place to spend the day in peaceful and tranquil surroundings. The main building was constructed from the original trees on site. They have an inviting gift shop managed by Marsha, with a variety of great souvenir items pertaining to nature that you can purchase for that special person in your life, and in the process you will be helping the Audubon Center to sustain itself financially. To all of you outdoor enthusiasts, make it a priority on your list of things to do and places to visit.

. . .

Note: Many of you may have viewed on New Hampshire Public Television the special that premiered on Sunday, October 4, at 8:00 p.m., a production entitled "Journey of the Broad-Winged Hawk." What a great story. Each year thousands of broad-winged hawks embark upon a 4,500-mile flight that takes them from their summer home in New Hampshire to their winter home in Ecuador and the Maquipucunu Reserve rich with wildlife. The TV special gave the viewers the opportunity to meet the people who follow the hawks' journey and have established connections with them.

38
Writing This Book

As Tim O'Brien states in his seminal story collection about his Vietnam experience, *The Things They Carried*, "Often in a true war story there is not even a point, or else the point doesn't hit you until twenty years later, in your sleep, and you wake up and shake your wife and start telling the story to her, except when you get to the end you've forgotten the point again. And then for a long time you lie there watching the story happen in your head. You listen to your wife's breathing. The war's over. You close your eyes. You take a feeble swipe at the dark and think, Christ, what's the *point*?"

I found more truth in this single book than in many of the nonfiction war stories I have read. Sometimes it is hard to convey a truth through the hard line of facts sans a story line—for one must have a story, a gripping yarn, an emotional hook to draw the reader in and keep him or her there. Perhaps more important than a clear ending or beginning, the story in the middle must be compelling, confusing, emotional, raw, dangerous, cruel, mean, courageous, wounding, taut like a ropy muscle in an angry person's neck. Sometimes I like to think of my story, this story, as simply a clothesline strung temporarily between two points—two trees, a tree and a back porch, a town in New Hampshire and an outpost in the desert, so to speak, and the clothes strung on the line—the story—written and displayed in sometimes discreet parts but in order, that is, all the socks hung together in a row and so forth, and sometimes not, with clothes strung as they are pulled from the laundry basket, with the presence of the wearer still embedded—a piece of underwear, a pair of pants, a shirt, a handkerchief, a baby's bib—parts strung out of order and as they are drawn by the hand that clips them to the line. Life unfolds in us that way sometimes, many times, repeatedly, and we later piece together the entire assemblage into a single outfit—or in my case, a single life story enclosed between the covers of a book.

Some may say my story is crazy and out of vogue with what's expected, what sells on someone else's best-seller list. But that is not the point of this. If you think it is, then you have failed as a reader to grasp the deeper intent, the one that stares you in the face and does not blink, wince, whine, or complain, the one that lets you assemble and reassemble this montage of my life, pieces really, between points beginning somewhere and ending who knows where, in any fashion that you wish. It even allows you to fill in the blanks between space and time; go ahead, take what is here, all that I have, and make a new story, adding, deleting, subtracting, and straightening out the clothes on my line and yours. Remember, as Tim O'Brien did, that the things you carry with you there and back again are what make the clothes hang straight or crooked or somewhere in between . . . the arrangement is really up to you and therein lays the truth of your story . . . and mine.

39

Recap

I am Robert Vallieres, and I wanted to be a career soldier ever since I can remember. But that did not happen; my career was cut short by an injury sustained in wartime but not on the field of battle, not outside the wire but by "friendly fire," material handling gone awry, and my head paid the price, as well as my heart and health.

I joined up right out of high school and was told I was accepted under the delayed enlistment program. I graduated from high school in June 1981 and entered the army in September 1982. I went to Fort Leonard Wood in Missouri for basic training, then to Fort Belvoir in Fairfax County, Virginia, to attend cartographic engineering school. I graduated in a few months and was assigned to Fort Bragg, North Carolina. I married my girlfriend, Carol St. Onge, that same year and she moved to North Carolina from northern New Hampshire with me. Fayetteville, North Carolina, became our new home.

Army life suited me, and my assignment while at Bragg included a stint mapping out endangered species habitat. A foreshadowing, I suppose, of my current volunteer work with birds. The bird habitat I mapped was for the red-cockaded woodpecker. I knew hardly anything about this bird and did not care about it back then. I can't recall if I ever saw one, but I knew how to identify their nesting trees.

When reenlistment came up I signed on again for another four years and was reassigned to Fort Shafter in Hawaii. Carol came with me. That was around 1986. While I was there, during a routine physical exam, the doctor noticed something not quite right with my heart and ordered further tests. Tests confirmed that I had an enlargement of my left ventricle, but I was told not to worry about it, that it would not prevent me from applying to Airborne School at Fort Benning in Georgia.

So I didn't worry. Life went along and I was preparing to leave Fort Shafter for Fort Benning in the early summer of 1990 when all hell broke loose in the Middle East. War was declared later that summer, in August, and everything changed for me and all the soldiers. We were told we would be deployed to the Middle East—Saudi Arabia probably but maybe Kuwait. I worried about my heart condition but was told by the docs that there was simply no time for any of them to consider writing up and defending a medical waiver to allow me to stay stateside on such short notice. I was given the medical equivalent of a thumbs-up and was added to the deployment roster.

So I was sent back to Fort Bragg and mobilized with the 175th Army Engineers, part of the 18th Airborne Corps, in Iraq during Operation Desert Shield/Storm. I was slotted in an E5 position with no promotion, so I remained an E4 in an E5 command spot. This happens in the army a lot. I headed to the desert with little or no time to prepare.

I got there and it was hot and dusty and flat. We wore desert camouflage and slept in tents. We were issued dust masks and bioweapons gas masks. Scuds went off all night long, not hitting anything really. I remember feeling displaced, yanked from one life into another with little to no preparation. I worried about my heart, my wife, me in this part of the world called the cradle of Christianity, except I was in Saudi, the headquarters of the Islamic faith. Women, bound head to toe in black cloth with a mysterious floating gate, just added to the weirdness of the place. I know that's not PC, but that is how it hit me . . . weird. So hot, colorless, and flat, with these shadowy figures in black moving as if they were spectral shadows where there is no shade. Seemed like I had flown through a time warp and ended up in the fifth century, except for the cars and the oil wells and the war and Americans en masse here at this outpost, our base of operations, a Martian landscape missing water, trees, oxygen, and shadows that create shade, a contrast to light.

Here I made maps for the officers so they could plot and plan strategy and know where the enemy was or where they thought the enemy should be. One time, during lunch, General Norman "Stormin' Norman" Schwarzkopf dropped in the mess hall and gave us a pep talk and used one of my maps as a visual to show locations, explain strategy, and give us a sense of the lay of the land, and just to have something to wave around as he spoke. That day was a high point for me. I was proud of my accomplishments and of how far I had come, a regular guy from a small northern New Hampshire town where French was my first language and where my mom and dad split and in the end it all turned out all right for me and I joined the army. That day when the general showed up, I loved the army and my uniform more than words can describe, a proud American doing what my country called me to do. Now that I think of it, it may have been Thanksgiving Day 1990.

That whole country was very foreign to me, the entire mobilization surreal. One day I was saying good-bye to Carol in our home in Fayetteville, North Carolina, and the next day I was landing here on this parched earth where God began his creation. But I was a soldier, so I did what I was told, dangling a gas mask and carrying a water bottle. I looked almost like a hiker in New Hampshire except for the odd-shaped mask meant to protect us from inhaling biowarfare agents, the munitions hanging from my cartridge belt, and my gun, not the kind I would go hunting with. I often wondered what would happen if the stuff, the biochemical warfare agent, landed on my arm. How would I protect my skin?

Later they deployed my unit to a waste dump in Kuwait to do some recon and map the area. We were told that this was a safe haven, that no one would bomb us in the dump, it not being a strategic target. The place reeked—indescribable, awful smells and toxic fumes. And we set up camp in the dump amid smoldering piles of humanity's castoffs, a waste stream that just lay on the ground and exposed us to its bubbling, burbling caldera of smoke, ash, and burnt sand. If hell were to come to earth, this is the place that would be the devil's home. And here we were, American soldiers, put here because someone in the know thought it a good way to keep us safe while we mapped out the general area. We had to map a bunch of flat nothingness and then just keep on mapping it out.

It was during the sixth month I was there that my accident happened, and my life went from being the way I had always known it to something in the Twilight Zone. It reminded me of the mind-and body-numbing shock of our football team not winning that final game against our archrival during my senior year. Just before we lost we were in a state of heightened alert and potential elation, adrenaline rushing and bodies tense, oozing camaraderie and the instinct to kill the ball, make the goal, and celebrate. But after the game ended and we realized that we had lost, we fell into a place of emotional pain and shock and physical nausea, bodies limp, crying without tears—some actually crying with tears.

The hit came from my left side, blindsided me, and knocked me to the ground. I grabbed at air to make the pain stop and then grabbed my head in my hands and fell sideways. My eye hurt and the entire left side of my head felt displaced, like it had moved a few degrees off the spinal pin that held it in place. I went from being able-bodied and doing my job, giving orders and joking with the guys, to being a fallen soldier, a victim of defeat, so to speak, crumpled up in pain, holding my head, and lying on the ground, whining and writhing in agony. At first I felt embarrassed, then angry, but the pain was so bad that all I could do was try not to cry, not to let go of consciousness, to get up to my knees and hold my head, try to stand. I thought my skull had been pierced, but when the medics arrived they said no. I thought I was bleeding, but the only red stuff dripping onto the sand was the Gatorade I had placed by my feet seconds before. I was put on a stretcher and carried off the field. Shit, I was hit by friendly fire, and not even from a firearm but from a young lieutenant who couldn't keep his attention on the task at hand long enough not to hit me with the wooden beam tossed off the back of a cargo truck. It hit me so solidly, as solidly as any projectile, that all I can be thankful for now is that the end that hit me was blunt and just missed piercing my skull and taking out my left eye by a hair's breadth.

Of course I felt terrible, embarrassed and weak at being hurt in a noncombat situation. Do you know what that feels like? It feels like you failed your guys and you failed yourself and you failed your country. To be hurt by a wooden beam flying through the air, a beam meant for some facility's construction on some Saudi-American construction project, was about the most embarrassing and worst circumstance I could imagine being in. I was just useless after that, always had headaches, and felt like I was complaining and whining about the pain all the time. But it was so bad I had to put myself in sick bay, and then I would throw up and feel like I wanted to tear into my head to stop the pain. I was also diagnosed with chronic neck contusions, and my neck never seemed to turn right after the whack in the head. I guess I was lucky that the beam missed my left eye by about a quarter inch. But I did not feel lucky at the time. I felt like a failure, angry and helpless because I could not make the beam hitting me in the head go away. It happened and I was a noncombat casualty and I had hardly been in a war zone at all. I was furious at the young lieutenant and furious at the way that it happened to me and that I could not go back and change it, just like I could never go back and win that last high school football game, no matter how much I replayed that touchdown missed by my teammate. I could not change the beam hitting me in the face as I turned to take the handoff from that damn punk officer.

Then came heart pain, constant and palpable. I tried to ignore it, downplaying it because my head hurt so much in comparison. Everything now felt hard to me, stress filled and pain ridden, so I didn't think much about my heart until I collapsed one day and could hardly catch my breath. I hurt in my chest and in my head and in my heart. Life hurt there in the desert sun. I lay on the ground, clutching my chest, feeling life seep out of me, ooze onto the sand, and then disappear underneath, seeking cool and shade. I must have passed out, because the next time I opened my eyes a doctor was above me, picking open my eyes, first one, then the other, and pulling the bottom lids down to look at the inside skin.

I was sent to a mobile medical tent and hooked up to an IV. My prognosis was not good. My heart was enlarged by an aortic aneurysm, a bulge somewhere in the left ventricle. It was the same disorder diagnosed back at Fort Shafter just before I was to attend Airborne School at Fort Benning. And I'd been mobilized anyway, sent here, bad heart and all. Now I was going home because of it or because of my head wound, or both. Everything just hurt and I lay there flat on my back, all hooked up to an IV.

A few days later I was medevaced offshore to the hospital ship USNS *Comfort*, a navy vessel set up to take on the casualties of war, not discriminating between combat-inflicted and noncombat wounds. When all was said and done, I was just glad to be on that ship and away from the parched and hostile heat. I wondered how Jesus could have stood it in this place that reeked to me of desolation and lack of water, shade, air full of oxygen, and the color green, a land abandoned by the rain.

That was then and this is now. I can't remember all the facts about my medical treatment after being sent back to the states. As I think back, Dacron mended my heart over here in the States at Walter Reed, and my head trauma was beginning to ease but still sputtering away. Then my rehab began. I don't remember much about that except docs telling me how I should feel and how I shouldn't feel and what I should and shouldn't do, or could do, or would never do. One thing is certain; I would never be a retired soldier. That hurt worst of all.

Carol was my lifeline and saving grace. She helped me through everything, even helping reconstruct my army career after it was lost on paper in some fire over in Saudi. I wonder still how the army could have lost me over there when I enlisted over here. Fire does strange things with paper and lives, I guess, and the army administration just couldn't find my records over here after that.

What I do remember about the rehab was that it was a strange process, with doctors, therapists, psychologists, and psychiatrists analyzing, diagnosing, and prescribing—but all of it from their external point of view. None of them were inside my body, my head, and my heart. What I found was that they really didn't know how to help me. The advice and pills they gave out made sense clinically to them but didn't really help me in the way I needed help. Anxiety and fear would overtake me and then the downward spiral of pain, remorse, anger, and guilt that I could not get better.

Then I attended school, which gave me an intellectual outlet where I could express some of my frustration and anger in a more creative way. I have a gift for drawing and expressing myself in words, and school gave me outlet for this. I learned a lot, gained self-confidence, and received my BA degree in drawing and illustration in May 2000 from Notre Dame College in Manchester, New Hampshire.

After that, I wondered what my next pursuit would be. I felt fairly certain that it would not be more of the same therapy, even though I was still struggling with depression, seizures, exhaustion, and very dark thoughts of suicide. I needed to find something of value that was outside myself but offered me sustaining interest on the inside, a love of something tangible that I could work with and relate to from my deepest being.

I was lucky because I found it in an ad for a birding trip. I was an outdoorsman and loved to fish but never considered looking at birds, never paid any attention to anything but the fish in the lake. But as soon as I went on this trip I was hooked! Birds found in me a place where no pills, therapies, or psychoanalysis could possibly go. All the advice the practitioners had given me was like a Band-Aid to dress a very deep and almost mortal wound and seemed to come from their perspective not mine. The birds simply walked into my heart and mind and, without judgment, perspective, criticism, or advice on what does and doesn't work, or should or shouldn't work, gave me back my life and my reason for being; they instilled in me hope, beauty, and excitement at a new discovery. Birds are right here and now, they are not in the future and they are not in the past. They are in the present moment, and the moment of discovery depends on the specific circumstance only—where you see them and what you notice when you see them. There is no good or bad, right or wrong, no needing to figure out the future. There is no forecast that my future is better or worse than it is right now. The birds don't care, and I don't either, as we exist only in the moment, right here and right now.

So bird watching is self-validating and self-healing, self-recuperative and self-redemptive. It's between you and the bird, or birds, and no one else, as to how you experience your time with them. And when your time with them is done, you walk down off the mountain without someone else's voice in your brain echoing solutions to your problems through the filter of their own perspective.

Birds rescue you from that and start building your confidence back up to get you out of your stuck place. They help you value yourself and your success as a human being, and your self-esteem begins to rekindle inside your sick heart and hurting head. For me, they bring forward a capability that stresses what I can do over what I cannot do. They give me my life force back and allow me to respect myself and my disability—and also my therapist's efforts at trying to help. No one can get inside your skin and be you (you need to claim that for yourself); what I learned from the birds is that it's okay for others to try, but only if you try harder to find in yourself where your new walk of life lies. And I hope, for me, it's where the birds are flying free or where they are caged and wounded and in need of a friend, a helper, a sympathetic soul.

In the end, birds have opened up the possibility for me to see myself differently and to see the world in which I exist differently. I must see both of these in order to see where and how I fit into the world now.

As a result of my work with birds, I have been written up numerous times in the New Hampshire Audubon newsletter, have had my photos of birds printed in local newspapers, and was lucky enough to be included in a film detailing the migration of the broad-winged hawks from New Hampshire to their wintering grounds in Ecuador. My most satisfying and emotional moment came, though, when I was chosen as the volunteer of the year by Volunteer NH. I am just a plain and ordinary guy who wanted to be a career soldier, married the woman I most loved in the world, was deployed during wartime to foreign lands, was diagnosed with a heart defect, and suffered a head injury. All of this combined to put me on an unexpected path, one that required me to heal and be healed, to accept that my goals would not be realized the way I had planned them out, to suffer and find a way out of my suffering, to try something I had never tried, and to realize that stepping out of my normal mold and into a new and untried walk has brought out in me a gentler, less angry, more creative and fulfilled human being. It's not that the pain is gone or that the depression has disappeared or that my heart beats stronger or that my mind is healed to near perfection. No, that's not it at all. I have learned to be grateful for my life, for the opportunities that have opened up for me and for new ones that await me. But most of all, I have learned to lean on those whom I love most—my wife and my son. They are the blessing bestowed on me from God above. To them, I am not the burden that I thought I was but simply the husband and the father. Love is stronger than my wounds, than my hurt, than my wanting it all to have turned out differently. It is what it is, and I am who I am, it's that simple, it's that real, and it's that way no matter how much I wish it wasn't. Wounds, by making us less than the perfect being we assumed we were before the wounding, can actually make us better by making us try harder to do the simple things we always took for granted, by making us more sensitive and compassionate toward others, instilling patience where there was none, a deeper and more abiding love for self and others close to us, and a sense of gratitude unrealized before things inside or outside our bodies malfunctioned or were lost forever. Wounds remind us of how vulnerable, fragile, and ephemeral our bodies can be. I have learned that every day is a blessing from above and that I need to stop and give thanks to God for what I have and not complain about what I don't have, no longer have, and can never get back.

As the saying goes, as one door closes, another opens. And I have cracked wide my new door and marched straight ahead into my new adventures. To that end, I and my coauthor have put together a plan to turn what I have done on my own into a blueprint for using birds in the therapy realm for all who are wounded and hurting, who do not know where to turn or what their next best step may be. We hope to implement a program that will give other Wounded Warriors the help I found in my avian adventures. Birds are a veritable feast of fascinating, unpredictable, and breathtaking movement that defies our ability to capture or control it. Perhaps that is what draws us to them: they represent the untamed wild in ourselves, allow us to overcome what limits us, to soar with them over mountaintops, and to skim across ocean waves. The program will tap into our connections with birds both near and far and will allow Wounded Warriors to experience the sense of mystery, magic, and devotion that birders feel for their feathered friends.

It's been twenty years since my injury. How do I ever get back those lost years? Not totally lost, but the memories are lost or, rather, not remembered right. I'm confused about that time after rehab when I was sent home to New Hampshire to live out the rest of my life with my wife and baby on the way. I don't remember the feelings I had when I walked through the door of my home for the first time after being discharged. Was I happy to be home, here in New Hampshire and not at Fort Bragg? Was I happy to have Carol by my side? Did I realize she was pregnant? I can't recall the exact moment of my son's birth; I just know that the day he was born, I had crippling pain in my head and my heart. My neck never stopped hurting. I remember wanting to die and live in the same breath. Should I shoot myself, take pills, step in front of a truck going down the highway, or jump off a cliff?

My docs chalk it all up to my injury. I don't even see in complete images sometimes. There's a medical name for that, but I've given up on the medical jargon. All I know is how I feel and how I don't feel, what I see and how I see it. Sounds simple but it really isn't. I play a constant fill-in-the-blanks game that I know will never have the outcome the docs want. I will never heal the way they want me to, and I will never go back to the way I was. Even twenty years later, I still suffer seizures, visual blanks, chronic tiredness, and headaches that seize any moment to pry open my head with thunder and lightning, along with just plain lack of stamina.

Birding helps me, though, with its requirements for attention to detail, singular focus, and patience, even as anger ebbs and flows like an AC/DC current in me. I wonder, as I sit in nature, if my memory of things is more selective, if I do it on purpose, or if it's really a result of my injury. Perhaps I've chosen to forget, not wanting to go back and relive the hot and desperately dry landscape where pain and trauma met in me and ended my career, my life changing with a quick toss and crack in the head. However that all happened back then, it sent me into a new place in life where birds matter more than all that stuff that came before. Stuff like puking my guts out on the desert sand, constant pain and writhing, sleeplessness, seizures, lack of purpose, depression, anger, and coiling and uncoiling thoughts of suicide.

I stayed married to my wife, whom I love most in the world and who gave me a son whom I love most in the world as well. I went to college, remained true to my faith, and prayed. And I found grace in birds. The birds gave me back a sense of purpose in this world where I was imprisoned. Especially the peregrines I watch in the wild and the eagles and owls I rehab in cages. I understand the wild bird injured and caged, perhaps never to take flight again. I look into the eyes of the untamed and proud birds, now impaired, and see myself looking out—stripped of dignity, having lost a wing, a foot, a leg, or an eye, or worse, their memory of flying or their ability to fly. I look at them behind bars, boxed in but retaining a vital life force, perhaps in the same way as I have, accepting that they can still play a purposeful role in life, showing others how it is to live differently.

Like the caged birds who test their wings daily even though one or both don't work anymore, I test myself, push myself a bit more each time I hike, observe, take down notes, think, ask questions, see what's at my feet as well as what's up on the ledge or high in the sky. I release myself to that "lightness of being" sensation as I fly on the wing with the birds, in cages or not, but especially with the peregrines, lifted up despite the press of gravity on my body. I write now and read. I draw and sketch and write poetry. I take pictures of birds, buildings, landscapes, and clouds. I'm not afraid to cry when I think of my son or of my wife's steadfastness and selflessness, her abiding commitment to me. I understand that as one door closes, another opens—but not automatically, and not without trial and error, lots of prayers, and stark raving honest introspection and self-reflection. Doors open, creating the space to move through to the other side, but it is up to you to walk the walk and end up on the other side. It is not the door that creates the opportunity but the space the door affords once opened. Closed doors afford a solid constraint; the door needs to be opened to create the opportunity. Conflict is inevitable, and sustained injury is an outcome of conflict, but it's how we respond that makes the difference.

The peregrine's lair is the home of my self-awakening and is as important to me as a symbol of freedom and unfettered movement as are the injured, once wild birds I care for in cages, constrained in freedom and movement, never to be released into the wild again. I feel deeply for them, especially for the eagles and other raptors that will never again fly over the weathered crevices and cliffs, never soar over oceans and fields, searching for prey, mates, the next perching spot, never again to fledge their young. They now depend on me to carry them on my arm, drop food in their trays, and clean their four-walled, single-roofed homes, making sure the dead trees used for perches are sturdy and strong. We all carry limitations within us—made, perceived, and acquired. How we live with them is how we make a difference in life. How we treat others with impairments, including birds, is a sign of our humanity, our dignity, our ability to love and take care of the things easily broken and left forgotten in a world imperfectly perfect, the world we call home station. God gives to each of us our own gifts and crosses to bear. Let us be to each other the grace of his gifts.

The war is long over. I went to war and I came back. I am Robert C. Vallieres. I am alive. I am here. I love my family. I embrace the life that God has given me. I'm injured inside where nobody can see the hurt. I work with birds. They know how it is with me. They and God heal me from my heart to my head. God gave me life. Birds saved my life. I live my life through them, with them, in them. Every day I wake up and walk my dream of a thousand paths, all leading me home to God, birds, and myself. My journey has included misery and near death, but I found a way toward healing and recovering—never completely healed and recovered—for what I am professing is an ongoing transfiguration or metamorphosis into life and learning. And it will not end. It will continue until I'm called home to heaven. I do not write this story because I have an answer. I write it because I have a voice, a story of healing grace, perhaps a message of hope to offer to others. I have no answers, only a process that I freely offer up. I take my long, slow drink of it every day like others do their glass of juice, cup of coffee, slug of Coke, or jigger of gin, depression, and misery.

What I've learned is that the things we carry with us can work either for us or against us. Like the soldiers in the casualty charts printed in newspapers and magazines and now on web pages, I could have been counted as one of the dead, but instead, I'm counted among the wounded. Now it's up to me to keep moving forward, living life beyond the injury, making the things I carry lighter, more meaningful, and more significant. I see my experience not as a burden to bear, an inglorious injury that left me disabled, left me with invisible wounds to my body, mind, spirit, and emotions, but as an opportunity to share with others and to offer help to them. To allow each and every military member who was left less whole after going to war than before an opportunity to help him- or herself through introducing birds into their lives. It's a wonderful modality that can be partaken of right where you are, whenever you choose, and in whatever physical space you find yourself. Watching birds is a "mind thing" where the object contributes to your senses in many ways—through sight, sound, color, movement, and internal processing. How you perceive the bird and what it means to you is a direct and very personal experience, without the need for interpretation, judgment, or analysis. There is no feedback loop, no right or wrong, no interpretive clinical diagnosis or outcome, just you, the birds, and your brain, heart, and soul.

As a dear friend and colleague, Dr. Fredric Abramson, says, "I can visualize the process [of bird watching] somewhat for [those who are] brain injured, though clearly not from their perspective." That is it, then, in a concise, airtight statement. No one can tell you what you are seeing when viewing birds. It's all up to you—to watch them, write about them, study them, take pictures of them, sketch them, listen to their songs, take them into your mind, and let them come out through your heart, where self-authentication happens and healing begins and recovery continues.

Jesus said, "Look at the birds of the air: they neither sow nor reap nor gather into barns, and yet your heavenly Father feeds them. Are you not of more value than they?" Think what the gift of birds can do for you, your family, your awakening to your new walk in life, a road less traveled but shared. On the wing and all around you, birds are there, from backyards and city streets to hospital windowsills and high mountaintops to lakes and rivers, oceans, and every single nook and cranny in between. They can be found in books, museums, art, music, song, and dance and in the very soul of each of us who understands flights of fancy and knows that hope is that thing with feathers that perches in the soul. The Belle of Amherst did, and why not us?

I have found my new walk, and writing this story is another chapter in my becoming Robert *Abled*, not Robert *Disabled*. As Robert Frost challenges us, dare to take the road less traveled and truly experience making a difference—in your own world and in the world outside you. Similarly, Henry David Thoreau encouraged us 150 years ago to find, and then march to, our own drum beat. Utilize what you have and caretake with dignity and grace those parts that are less than whole or that no longer function, respond to, or grasp things the way they once did. Let yourself experience a new outlook, a new hobby, a renewal of self in nature, a healing connection with the birds, soaring above the critical mass. Hold on and experience your very own self-authenticating, self-interpreting, and self-healing recovery on the wing!

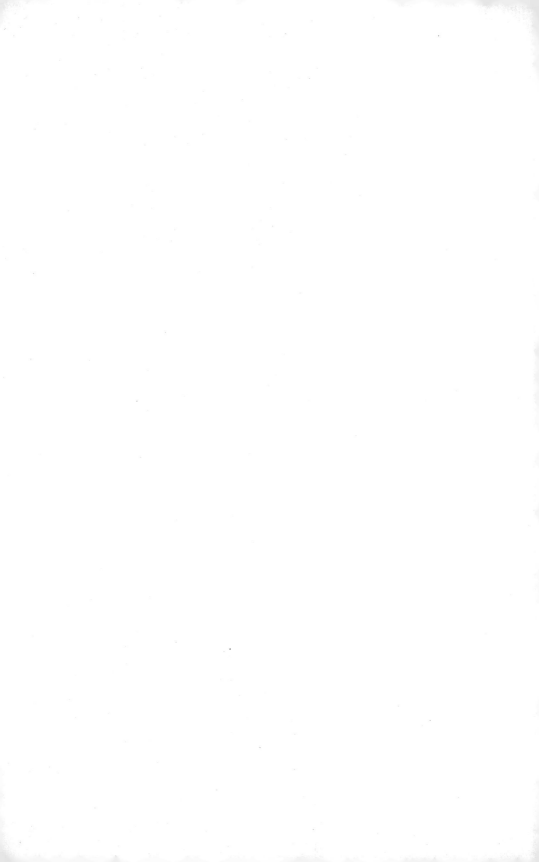